TASHLULTUM LEVY

The Ruth Diet

Turning Back Time in 30 Days

Contents

I

The Path to Wellness: Ruth's Metaphoric Journey of Transformation

1

Reading The Book of Ruth

The Book of Ruth is a short yet powerful book in the Bible, comprising only four chapters. If you want to read it over the course of a month (30 days), you could evenly distribute it over weeks, allowing time to ponder the message and apply it to your life. Here's a suggested reading schedule:

Week 1 (Days 1-7)

- Day 1: **Introduction** - Read initial summaries, introductions, or commentaries to familiarize yourself with the story of Ruth.
- Day 2-4: **Ruth Chapter 1** - Divide the chapter into three parts and read a part each day.
- Day 5-7: **Reflection and Study** - Reflect on the lessons learned from Chapter 1. You may want to re-read certain verses, jot down thoughts, or discuss insights with others.

Week 2 (Days 8-14)

- Day 8-10: **Ruth Chapter 2** - Divide the chapter into three parts and read a part each day.
- Day 11-14: **Reflection and Study** - Reflect on the themes from Chapter 2. This could include writing down thoughts, studying deeper with

commentaries, or sharing insights in a group.

Week 3 (Days 15-21)

- Day 15-17: **Ruth Chapter 3** - Divide the chapter into three parts and read a part each day.
- Day 18-21: **Reflection and Study** - Reflect on Chapter 3. This could involve personal meditation, writing in a journal, or group discussion.

Week 4 (Days 22-28)

- Day 22-24: **Ruth Chapter 4** - Divide the chapter into three parts and read a part each day.
- Day 25-28: **Reflection and Study** - Reflect deeply on the themes and insights from Chapter 4. Write your thoughts, discuss them, or deep dive into commentaries for better understanding.

Week 5 (Days 29-30)

- Day 29-30: **Overall Reflection and Review** - Read the Book of Ruth as a whole, connect the chapters, and reflect on the overarching messages and themes. This is a time for a final review and to personally relate to the story.

This schedule allows you to gradually absorb the story, ponder its message, and relate it to your own life experiences, providing a rich and rewarding study of the Book of Ruth.

2

The Path to Wellness: Ruth's Metaphoric Journey of Transformation

In our exploration of The Book of Ruth, the narrative takes on symbolic depth, paralleling a journey in pursuit of overall wellness and a healthier lifestyle.

Ruth signifies a soul ready to leave behind the familiar for a multitude of unknowns. Documented in Ruth's decision to follow Naomi, her mother-in-law, we witness the sacrifice of stepping away from old ways and venturing into unprecedented territory. This symbolizes the resolution we must make when we choose health and wellness over the seemingly comforting, but detrimental repertoire of unhealthy practices we've grown accustomed to.

Naomi symbolizes the wisdom of the ages, etched with the patina of time and experience. Her decision to return to her roots and the ways of her ancestors mirrors our own journey back to genuine nutrition — to grains, whole foods, and unprocessed nourishments provided by nature. It's a rediscovery of the fundamental truth that simplicity and purity in our diet can serve as a healing balm against the afflictions triggered by a world saturated with artificiality and excess.

And then, there is Boaz — a metaphor for the richness of a healthier lifestyle that cherishes and respects the bounty of the land. Boaz, embodying the proverbial land of 'milk and honey,' encourages a lifestyle that relishes homegrown, natural foods, in stark contrast to the consumption trends dictated by the modern world. This underscores our awakening towards the beauty of living off the land, appreciating its nutritious offerings, and rejecting the allure of unhealthy, processed foods.

This section of the book hence mirrors a transformative journey from old, unhealthy habits towards a rejuvenated existence nurtured by nutritious grains, fresh produce, and a deep affiliation with the natural world. It's a quest towards overall wellness, invigorated by the wisdom of the past and the gifts of the Earth, much like Ruth's journey alongside Naomi towards the land of Boaz.

3

Ruth - Leaving the Familiar Behind

Once upon a time, in the land of Moab, lived a young woman named Ruth. Her life, as she knew it, was about to drastically change. With the death of her husband, Ruth found herself at a crossroads—return to her native Moab to the family she had always known, or embark upon an uncertain journey with her mother-in-law, Naomi, to an alien land, Bethlehem.

Mirroring our dilemmas, when confronted with a path towards health and wellness, Ruth held the essence of a soul staring into the myriad unknowns. As we often grapple with new diets or fitness routines, Ruth had to wrestle with her familiar versus the unfamiliar.

In an act of unequivocal commitment, Ruth told Naomi, "Where you go, I will go; where you lodge, I will lodge; your people shall be my people, and your God my God." These reverberating words signified her willingness to step away from her old ways, venturing boldly and bravely into an unprecedented life.

This symbolic narrative parallels the difficult resolution we often encounter when an unhealthy lifestyle that we're used to, although comforting, becomes detrimental to our health. At such turning points, just like Ruth, we are obliged to leave behind the familiarity and comfort of our unhealthy practices, embracing a challenging yet ultimately rewarding path towards health and wellness.

Craving change is not enough; Ruth teaches us the necessity of making tough decisions in our quest for self-improvement. Every step away from our previous unhealthy lifestyle, every salad chosen over junk food, every mile jogged instead of an evening on the couch, signifies our commitment to a healthier life, an echo of Ruth's courageous choice.

This is the beginning of a story marked by resolve, courage, and transformation; the dawn of Ruth's metaphoric journey towards wellness, and perhaps ours too.

4

Naomi - Guiding Wisdom and Ancestral Ways

As Ruth set foot on the path alongside her mother-in-law, they embarked on a journey cloaked in uncertainty, and yet, filled with potential. Naomi, grappling with her share of loss and sorrow, had decided to return to Bethlehem, to the ancestral roots that called to her with the promise of healing.

Naomi embodies the timeless wisdom and experience of generations past, never to be forgotten. In making her choice to reunite with her people's traditions, she finds solace in their age-old knowledge and ways of living. These ancestral connections mirror our journey from unhealthy lifestyles to the rediscovery of genuine nutrition, be it like the biblical manna, a gift from nature that heals and nourishes.

Through Naomi's wisdom, we find inspiration to embrace the grains, whole foods, and unprocessed sustenance that nature provides. The simplicity and purity of our ancestors' diet serve as a balm against the afflictions stemming from a world inundated with artificiality and excess. This rediscovery connects one's essence to the very core of their being, the source of true healing.

Ruth observed and learned from Naomi, embracing the ways of her mother-in-law and her community. In doing so, she becomes the personification of adaptability, courage, and receptiveness—traits that we must emulate on our own pursuit of wellness.

The bond between Ruth and Naomi illustrates the transformative power of tapping into the wisdom of the ages. The nurturing guidance afforded by time-tested knowledge steers one through a journey of self-discovery and renewed vitality, propelling us towards a healthier life infused with ancestral wisdom.

II

Ruth: Leaving The Familiar Behind

5

Ruth - Unfamiliar Paths

As dawn broke over the foreign lands of Bethlehem, Ruth felt the magnitude of her decision. Leaving the familiar had never been an easy task, but it was a step she had been resolute in taking.

Just like the daunting prospect of discarding old habits, Ruth was venturing out of her comfort zone. However, it was not only about leaving the familiarity of Moab behind, but it was an embrace of a journey towards resilience, growth, and ultimately, transformation.

Ruth was facing the unknown, much like we do when we make tough decisions for our wellness. Coming from a world seeped in unhealthy practices and comforting routines, the dominance of the unknown can sometimes cause doubt and fear. However, Ruth invited the challenge, her heart resolute in the pursuit of a better future.

Each day in Bethlehem presented Ruth with new experiences and challenges to overcome. Every grain harvested, every Perek (melodious song of praise) learned, became a step towards integrating into this new world. These experiences symbolize our own journey when we consciously opt to incorporate healthier practices into our life.

By challenging the comforting familiarity of her past life and embracing the unpredictability of her new journey, Ruth teaches us a valuable lesson. Even amid the discomfort that comes with transformation, one must forge on, for the path to wellness often lies in leaving behind the familiarity of the detrimental and stepping courageously towards the unfamiliar promise of well-being.

Much like Ruth's experience on the roads of Bethlehem, our journey to wellness may not be easy. Yet, it is rightfully ours to undertake, fortified by the knowledge that on this path lies a promise for a healthier, more vibrant life.

6

The Sacrifices Along the Path

Departing from the familiar encompasses a series of sacrifices, and Ruth's journey was no exception. She traded comfort for challenge, and certainty for ambiguity. Ruth's choices symbolize the personal sacrifices required when one makes wellness a life priority.

Just as Ruth gave up the comforts of Moab, we too need to forsake the comforting allure of unhealthy meals, sedentary lifestyles, and harmful habits. This doesn't come easy; it demands effort, persistence, and a resilient will. In many ways, these sacrifices are an echo of Ruth's journey – uncomfortable but indispensable for the ultimate reward.

The path towards wellness confronts us with choices that stretch our resilience, echoing Ruth's decision to stick with Naomi and work hard in the fields for their sustenance. It was an echo of the painstaking journey towards achieving a healthier body and mind – from the sweat of intense workouts to the restraint needed to avoid detrimental consumptions.

Ruth's narrative builds the understanding that sacrifices are integral to any transformational journey. Such personal sacrifices for the sake of health and wellness might seem overwhelming initially, similar to the estrangement and hardship Ruth faced.

However, viewing Ruth's journey through the wellness prism, we realize that these sacrifices aren't just about giving up, they are about engaging in the process of redefining our lives. Each sacrifice creates space for new experiences and learnings, marking a growth pattern that constructs a healthier and fulfilling life.

7

The Transformation's Trials and Triumphs

Instigating change in life requires sacrifices — Ruth understood this too well. In leaving behind her familiar land of Moab, she confronted the trials one faces while prioritizing health and wellness.

Ruth's sacrifices mirrored ours when we choose to step away from convenience and indulgence to embrace a lifestyle founded on self-care and discipline. Like the withdrawal from a leisurely Moabite lifestyle, we too, move away from the seemingly secure comfort of our old habits, trading it for potential growth and wellness on a path mainly dictated by uncertainties.

The journey might seem arduous, just as Ruth's sojourn to an alien land, working tirelessly in the fields, giving her sweat and effort in hopes of a better future. Likewise, we are often confronted with demanding workouts and disciplined diets. The transformation of fitness and wellness rarely comes without discomfort; they demand perseverance, much like Ruth's unwavering commitment to her new life.

But amidst these trials arise moments of triumph, instances where we feel empowered and invigorated. Ruth found her moments in gathering grains, providing for Naomi, and her eventual acceptance within the Bethlehem community. Similarly, our victories may appear in different forms, as every pound lost to healthful eating, every improved mile timing, or every time we choose a wholesome meal over fast food.

Through Ruth's journey, we learn that personal sacrifices are indeed part of any transformational journey towards health and wellness. These trials, daunting as they may be, ultimately aid in growth, leading us, much like Ruth, towards a fulfilling, rewarding path of wellness and healthier life.

III

Naomi: Wisdom and Ancestral Ways

8

Ancestral Traditions Illuminated Through Naomi

Naomi, an emblem of time-honored wisdom and ancestral traditions, generously shared her knowledge with Ruth, as she made her way through her wellness journey in the land of Bethlehem. As Ruth learns to appreciate her new world, the lessons imparted by Naomi are influential for Ruth's growth and success.

Through the narrative of Naomi, we're reminded of the benefits of returning to the roots of indigenous wisdom. Just like how ancestral knowledge nourishes the soul, it also fosters a foundation for holistic living. Embracing the concepts presented by Naomi, such as weaving a healthier relationship with the natural world, we too can channel the same time-honored wisdom.

Naomi alludes to the importance of recognizing the values of ancestral traditions, especially those related to the cultivation of a fulfilled life. These practices often revolve around fundamental ideals, such as a deeper connection with the Earth and its gifts, a focus on communal support, and a life anchored in vibrant spiritual fitness.

The teachings and guidance of Naomi offer a deeper understanding of how ancient wisdom can be linked to achieving a strong mind-body balance. In adopting these ancestral principles, we embark on a path to wellness that goes beyond physical health. It serves as a reminder that reclaiming this long-lasting wisdom positively impacts our lives in ways that modern healthcare often cannot achieve alone.

9

The Wholesome Path of Ancestral Nutrition: Ruth's Gradual Embrace of a New Lifestyle

Ruth's progression mirrors our path towards wellness, initially stumbling upon a field of natural grains, representing a healthier lifestyle. At first, she isn't ready to wholly embrace the change epitomized by Boaz, even though her newfound nourishment sets her on a new path. The lessons from Naomi's wisdom and ancestral ways extend beyond the past; they draw compelling parallels to our modern journey towards a healthier and more fulfilling life. Naomi's guidance resonates within the realm of wholesome nutrition, aiding Ruth in embracing a natural and balanced lifestyle.

In the same vein, we can learn from these time-honored principles by returning to the basics and rediscovering the sustenance provided by nature. Before marrying the healthy lifestyle symbolized by Boaz, Ruth starts by gleaning from the field of natural grains. By selecting whole, unprocessed foods and harnessing the inherent healing properties found in plants and ancient grains, we journey back to what nurtured generations before us.

Naomi's understanding of ancestral nutrition highlights the importance of preserved wisdom, as it connects us to the essence of natural sustenance, something often overlooked in a world of convenience and artificiality.

Emulating that simplicity in our modern lives can bring us closer to the state of balance and harmony embodied by our ancestors.

To follow in the footsteps of Ruth, who learned from Naomi, we can rekindle our relationship with earth-based wisdom. Gradually, like Ruth among the gleaned grains, we can attune our consumption habits to the rhythm of nature, eventually embracing a committed lifestyle that promotes our physical, mental, and spiritual well-being.

10

The Healing Power of Simplicity and Purity in Our Diet: Purging the Unwanted

Drawing further insights from Naomi's wisdom and ancestral ways, it becomes clear that simplicity and purity in our diet can be instrumental in healing and nourishing our bodies. These principles serve as guiding lights on our wellness journey, much like the beacon of wisdom that Naomi was for Ruth.

Simplicity, in the context of diet, refers to a focus on natural, whole foods. It invites a way of eating that prioritizes fresh produce, unprocessed grains, lean proteins, and healthy fats. This simplistic approach to nutrition aligns closely with how our ancestors ate, which largely avoided modern-day issues of processed food consumption.

Purity encapsulates the essence of eating foods as close to their natural state as possible. It rejects artificial additives, preservatives, and high levels of sodium and sugars that are often found in processed foods. By embracing pure, unadulterated foods, we provide our bodies with the nutrients they require for optimal functionality, fostering a more robust immune system and better overall health.

Ruth's journey includes the symbolic act of washing her face, representing thee act of purging impurities and unwanted elements from her body and life. This metaphorical cleanse aligns with embracing simplicity and purity in her diet, further emphasizing the importance of eliminating harmful substances from our nutrition.

Ruth's slow transformation reflects the wisdom of incorporating simplicity and purity in her diet. This gradual change shows us that achieving health and wellness doesn't require drastic measures but, instead, mindful choices, paced transitions, and sustainable practices, as suggested by Naomi's wisdom. With this understanding, we can confidently journey towards greater physical well-being while honoring the wisdom of our ancestors.

IV

Boaz as a Metaphor for a Wholesome Lifestyle

11

Nurturing the Land's Bounty and Honoring Dietary Law

In the unfolding story of Ruth's transformation and learning, Boaz represents the richness of a healthier lifestyle and the celebration of nature's abundant offerings. As Ruth begins to embrace the wisdom imparted by Naomi and the cleanliness that comes with obeying dietary laws, Boaz becomes an integral symbol of the authentic, holistic lifestyle Ruth aspires to attain.

Boaz's role in the narrative embodies a deep connection with the land and a reverence for its bounty. His dedication to nurturing nature's resources not only illustrates his personal commitment to living in harmony with the earth but also demonstrates respect for the dietary laws, seeing food as a divine gift to be honored and treated with care.

This obedience to God's dietary laws is not merely a restrictive practice but a conscious decision to honor our bodies as sacred vessels, feeding them with nutrients given to us by God's providence through nature. By adhering to these laws, Ruth combines her faith with her journey towards a healthier lifestyle.

The gradual shift in Ruth's life towards Boaz's metaphorical embodiment of optimal health highlights the importance of taking a patient, measured approach to our wellness journey. Just as Ruth required time to internalize the lessons from Naomi, adapt to new dietary habits, and adhere to the divine dietary laws, our personal transitions towards better health and well-being often require patience, persistence, and dedication.

As we learn from Ruth and Boaz, embarking on a path towards a healthier lifestyle means embracing and nurturing the land's bounty with gratitude and respect. By developing a profound connection with nature, we can fuel our bodies and minds with the vibrancy and richness that comes from living in accordance with earth's natural rhythms and God's sacred dietary laws.

12

The Contrast Between Natural, Homegrown Foods and Modern Consumption Trends

In our pursuit of a healthier lifestyle, exemplified by the bountiful metaphor of Boaz, we encounter the need to examine the striking contrast between natural, homegrown foods and modern-day consumption trends. By understanding these disparities, we can make more informed choices that support our wellness journey and deepen our connection with the earth.

Natural, homegrown foods are a testament to the simplicity and richness of nature's offerings. They are nurtured by sunlight, water, and fertile soil, embodying Boaz's principles of harmony with the earth. Consuming fresh, homegrown produce nourishes our bodies as nature intended, providing essential nutrients, vitamins, and minerals.

On the other hand, modern consumption trends often lean heavily on processed and convenience foods. While they might offer momentary satisfaction and ease, they tend to be laden with artificial additives, preservatives, excess salt, and sugars, detracting from the purity and integrity of our diet.

As we follow Ruth's journey, we learn the importance of seeking harmony with nature and paying mind to our connection with the land and its bounty. Her faithfulness to the dietary laws of God, as practiced by her ancestors, not only aligns her with natural, homegrown foods but also brings her great blessings. This reinforces the idea that honoring these dietary laws goes beyond mere obedience, leading us to healthier, more fulfilling lives.

A healthier lifestyle embraces the beauty and wisdom of our ancestors' way of living in alignment with nature. By consciously choosing to honor the tradition of natural, homegrown foods and adhering to divine dietary laws, we distance ourselves from destructive modern consumption trends and take significant strides towards a more nourished, wholesome life.

13

Embracing Natural, Homegrown Foods for a Richer Life

In this wellness journey, the marked transformation we seek is not just a rejection of unhealthy, processed foods, but also a radiant embrace of natural, homegrown foods. As the narrative continues, Boaz—represented as a metaphor for the healthier lifestyle—offers us a vivid reminder of vitality and wellbeing inherent in foods cultivated straight from Mother Earth.

Seemingly convenient, processed foods, disguise the stark reality of their nutritional deficiencies. High levels of sodium, sugars, unhealthy fats, as well as artificial preservatives and additives make up their composition, leading to gradual compromise of our health and wellbeing.

Drawing lessons from Ruth's steadfast adherence to the dietary laws of her ancestors reflects our journey towards optimal health. This journey implies not just a conscious shift in our dietary habits—letting go of processed food—but also celebrating our bodies as divine temples, deserving of pure and well-balanced nourishment.

Taking it further, the path we tread prompts us to not just consume, but also produce—grow our own food, just as Ruth's ancestors did. This connection to the land and the fruits it offers is an enriching, joyous experience, allowing us to embrace the wholesomeness that Boaz represents, enhancing our overall wellbeing.

This crucial shift in dietary habits, however, should not be mistaken as a call for rigid measures or self-deprivation. On the contrary, it is an invitation—a call to appreciate nature's bountiful generosity, nourishing our bodies with food, as was originally intended by God and as nature provides.

Standing firmly in our decision to reject processed foods and grow our own, mirroring Ruth's commitment to a healthier way of life, we take a significant stride towards experiencing the richness of a Boaz lifestyle.

V

The Journey of Transformation

14

Cordoning off Detrimental Habits for a Rejuvenated Existence

As we continue on this transformative journey inspired by The Book of Ruth, we recognize that change is an integral part of growth. This change involves identifying and cordoning off old, detrimental habits to make room for a rejuvenated existence brimming with wellness and vitality.

Much like Ruth, we are called upon to detach from practices that no longer serve our wellbeing. It is a process of excavating deep-rooted dietary habits embedded in convenience and instant gratification, replacing them with conscious choices that honor our bodies and the bountiful earth.

Cutting off from processed foods and embracing homegrown, natural foods is a transformative shift. It is a shift towards cultivating a direct connection with the land, valuing freshness, and prioritizing nutritional balance.

Embracing this change also prompts us to adopt a holistic view of wellness, understanding that a healthy lifestyle extends beyond just our plates. It involves fostering a positive mental state, engaging in regular physical activity, and indulging in restful sleep patterns while maintaining social connections.

This change may initially seem daunting or even overwhelming. Yet, it is essential to remember that the path of transformation, though fraught with challenges, reaps beautiful rewards, renewing us from within.

Drawing inspiration from Ruth, we learn that cordoning off detrimental habits is not a rejection of the past but a celebration of potential—a potential that nourishes, strengthens, and rejuvenates us on this journey toward wellness.

With each mindful choice, we echo Ruth's journey, stepping closer to a vibrant, rejuvenated existence, embracing the richness of a Boaz lifestyle.

15

The Transformation Journey Reflected in The Book of Ruth

The journey of transformation symbolized in The Book of Ruth unfolds as an enriching narrative filled with lessons on wellness and wholeness. We see Ruth, a Moabite widow, grow into a woman of strength, faith, and resilience, reflecting our profound journey toward a healthier lifestyle.

The Book of Ruth tells the story of Ruth's loyalty to Naomi, her adherence to the dietary laws of her ancestors, and her ultimate elevation in Boaz's fields. Much like our personal wellness journeys, Ruth faced challenges but remained committed to her true path.

Ruth's transformative journey acts as a guiding light for us as we seek to create healthier habits. Her devotion to natural and homegrown food reminds us of the essence of wellness: honoring our bodies, the very temples of life, by seeking sustenance from what nature abundantly offers.

One of the profound messages settling into our hearts is the necessity of mindfulness in everything we do, including our dietary choices. By consciously rejecting the processed and unhealthy, and choosing to nurture our bodies with homegrown, natural foods, we echo Ruth's journey.

Drawing strength from Ruth's narrative, we reaffirm our commitment to this transformative journey. This path may appear daunting at first glance, fraught as it is with sacrifices and lifestyle changes. Yet, as Ruth's story revealed, the ultimate rewards of well-being, peace, and prosperity are well worth the effort.

As Ruth blossomed in her transformation, so shall we in our journey, moving ever closer to achieving the harmony and wholeness embodied by Boaz.

16

Nourishing Life through Grains, Fresh Produce, and an Attachment with Nature

Tracing the path set out by Ruth in her transformative journey, the significance of nutritious grains, fresh produce, and a deep bond with nature emerges prominently. This chapter explores these crucial elements that further illuminate our path to wellness and wholeness.

Nutritious grains, integral to Ruth's diet, symbolize the sustenance and health benefits provided by nature. Rich in fiber, vitamins, and minerals, these grains offer essential nutrients that maintain our overall health. They represent a leap from processed to natural, reminding us of our roots on this journey toward wellness.

Fresh produce, harvested straight from the earth, provides us unmatched vitality and well-being, just as they did for Ruth. Each fruit and vegetable carries its unique health benefit, providing our bodies with necessary vitamins, antioxidants, and phytonutrients, reminding us to value and cherish nature's abundance.

The deeper significance of this journey lies not merely in the consumption of grains and fresh produce but more so in the process of their cultivation. Echoing Ruth's attachment with nature, tending to the land and reaping its fruits elevates our appreciation for the Earth's generosity. This connection with nature nurtures not only our bodies but also our minds and spirits, creating a holistic sense of health and well-being.

While navigating this transformative path, we come to respect and cherish the role of nutritious foods such as grains and fresh produce. In tandem, our bond with nature grows stronger, adding a spiritual layer to our journey, reminding us of Ruth's continuous attachment to the land.

With each conscious dietary choice and interaction with nature, we step closer to living our enriched, empowered existence, mirroring a Boaz lifestyle.

VI

Conclusion

17

Conclusion - The Quest Towards Holistic Wellness

As we close this section of our journey towards transformation, we reflect on the immense wisdom and inspiration that Ruth's narrative offers us. Charting a path from processing to natural, from convenience to consciousness, from detachment to deep connections, we steadily align more closely with a lifestyle that prioritizes holistic wellness and rejuvenation.

Emphasizing the role of nutritious grains and fresh produce, Ruth's story urges us to reimagine our diet not as a chore or obligation, but as an expression of our respect and gratitude for the Earth's abundance. Our move towards home-grown food tells a story of attachment with nature, reminiscent of Ruth's continued bond with the earth and its generous produce.

Similarly, veering away from detrimental habits to adopt healthier ones shines the spotlight on self-improvement and potential. The quest towards holistic wellness is far from a rejection of our previous ways but is instead an acceptance of a richer, rejuvenated existence that aligns with the Boaz lifestyle.

Much like Ruth, we learn that true transformation radiates from within, nourished by healthier lifestyle choices, proactive mental health care, and an unwavering commitment to physical wellness. Importantly, it also emphasizes the need to foster meaningful social connections that further enhance our life journey, mirroring the bonds Ruth cultivated on her path to transformation.

Reflecting on Ruth's equanimity in the face of obstacles, we learn that resilience and steadfastness transform challenges into stepping stones towards wellness. As we continue exploring the landscape of holistic wellness, each step becomes an echo of Ruth's journey, affirming our commitment to transformation and the quest towards holistic wellness.

18

Conclusion - Linking Ruth and Naomi's Journey to Boaz's Land with Our Pursuit of a Healthier Lifestyle

In closing, we link Ruth and Naomi's journey to Boaz's land with our own pursuit of a healthier lifestyle. Much like their steadfast devotion to one another and faith in forging a better life, we, too, embark on a path filled with challenges and triumphs toward elevating our overall well-being.

Ruth's unwavering loyalty to Naomi symbolizes the importance of support and encouragement in our own quests for transformation. By surrounding ourselves with loved ones who share our vision of wellness, resilience, and self-improvement, we find strength and motivation in our common goals.

As Ruth and Naomi journeyed on and ultimately prospered in Boaz's land, so do we as we immerse ourselves in the richness of holistic wellness. We establish conscious connections with nature, cultivate our passions, and foster meaningful relationships that fuel our emotional, mental, and physical growth.

The story of Ruth, while a testament to the might of personal transformation, also serves as a reminder that our wellness is not a solitary endeavor. Instead, it flourishes within a supportive community of individuals who inspire, uplift, and encourage one another.

In essence, our journey toward a healthier lifestyle is an ongoing, shared expedition of growth and fulfillment. Just as Ruth and Naomi forged their way to Boaz's land and carved a path of strength, sustenance, and solace, our pursuit of well-being draws us closer to the ideal of harmony, happiness, and wholeness.

19

Conclusion - Reconnecting with Our Roots and Harnessing Wisdom from the Past

As we navigate the concluding chapter of this transformative journey, one theme prominently surfaces, affirming its indispensable role – the necessity of reconnecting with our roots and harnessing wisdom from the past to promote health and wellness.

Much like Ruth and Naomi's journey, our pursuit of wellness is steeped in age-old wisdom, ancestral practices, and enduring principles that bind us to our roots and guide us toward a holistic lifestyle. This wisdom teaches us to embrace the bounties of nature, appreciate its healing power, and foster a profound respect that extends beyond our plates into our consciousness.

Our roots, embedded in the communal bond of sharing, teach us about the importance of nourishment, not just for our bodies but our souls and minds as well. They introduce us to the power of nutritious grains, fresh produce, and the timeless knowledge derived from our ancestors, which we incorporate into our modern lives to promote wellness.

As we journey on, we engrain these lessons of the past into our present, just as Ruth did years ago on her transformative journey. We incorporate these teachings into our daily practices, meticulously weaving them into the fabric of our lives.

In this transformation, we experience the joys of eating wholesome foods, connect deeper with the earth, strike a balance with nature, and most importantly, harmonize our physical, emotional, and spiritual well-being to tread successfully on this path to wellness.

Ultimately, it is clear that our journey towards wellness isn't a path forged ahead alone, but a collective effort of remembering our roots, learning from the wisdom of the past, and working together as a community towards a healthier, happier future.

VII

Introduction

20

An Introduction to 'The Ruth Diet'

As dawn breaks, casting its ethereal light on the world, you stir, awakened by a deep resolve within. Today marks your initiation into a transformative journey — the journey of 'The Ruth Diet'. This empowering venture is more than just a regimen; it's a call to reclaim vitality and rejuvenate your body and spirit within just 30 days.

At the core of The Ruth Diet lies a profound yet simple philosophy: a 100% liquid fast, designed to cleanse not just the body but also the mind. This holistic approach seeks to facilitate a deeper connection between body, mind, and soul, fostering harmony and balance throughout your being.

The journey may be challenging, keeping solid food at bay, but its rewards far outweigh the temporary trials. Through a thoughtful blend of nutritious, satiating liquids and empowering habits, you hope to restore balance and discover a healthful equilibrium.

You begin your mornings with a warm cup of detox tea, a simple concoction with the essence of rejuvenation. With each gentle sip, you imagine the infusion coursing through you, flushing out toxins and remnants of past indulgences.

As your day progresses, you keep your body replenished with an array of vibrant juices, rich vegetable broths, and hearty soups. Each glass or bowl is a testament to your commitment to this new chapter, a resolve mirrored in the vivid hues of the countless fruits and vegetables used to prepare your meals.

To enhance your experience, you integrate various mindfulness practices, such as meditation and deep-breathing exercises. Through these activities, you cultivate inner calmness and increase mental clarity, thus nurturing harmonious synergy between your body and mind.

The nights hold their own ritual. A warm glass of water with a squeeze of fresh lemon serves as your concluding routine. You fondly think of it as your moonlight cup, marking the end of yet another successful day of commitment.

The core of 'The Ruth Diet' isn't a rigorous demand on the self but rather a gentle invitation to reinvent the everyday. It's a promise to realign yourself with the rhythm of nature, an opportunity to mirror the ebbs and flows of natural life.

However, it's not just about cleansing the body. The Ruth Diet extends its deep, purifying ethos to the skin as well. Using natural treatments and consciously developed habits, you understand the essential link between wholesome nutrition and glowing skin. The goal isn't only to attain a younger appearance but to bring forth the inner radiance that defines true wellness.

This 30-day revitalizing journey won't be without its challenges. The path to redefining your dietary habits, and by extension, your life, is steep and might seem daunting. But you remain undeterred, as you know that your commitment to The Ruth Diet – to yourself, your happiness, your health – is a beacon guiding you forward, turning back the hands of time a little more with each passing day.

It's the dawn of your adventure into 'The Ruth Diet'. The journey to rejuvenation begins as you take the first step toward a healthier, refreshed tomorrow, defying the constraints of time one nourishing liquid meal at a time. As you embark on this transformative experience, you gain not only physical health benefits but also an enriched understanding of the interconnectedness between body, mind, and spirit, ultimately paving the way for a thriving, revitalized life.

21

Unlocking The Ruth Diet

Welcome, dear reader, to a transformative journey unlike any other – introducing The Ruth Diet, a pathway to rejuvenate your being, inside and out. Rooted in ancient wisdom, yet astoundingly relevant to our contemporary lives, The Ruth Diet brings to your table a refreshingly holistic approach to health and wellness.

The Ruth Diet, inspired by the lore of the indomitable Ruth, is more than just a dietary regimen. It is a comprehensive wellness program that marries time-tested wisdom with innovative practices to pave the way for a healthier, more vibrant you. Timeless and incredibly pertinent in today's world, it is designed to foster physical vitality, mental clarity, and spiritual serenity.

At the core of The Ruth Diet are three fundamental principles – rejuvenation, detoxification, and spiritual wellness. Each of these pillars is built upon the understanding that our body, mind, and spirit are intricately woven together, forming the extraordinary tapestry of human life.

As you journey along The Ruth Diet, you can expect a physical rejuvenation that manifests in increased vitality, radiant skin, and improved overall health. The detoxification component aims to cleanse your body from within, flushing out toxins and promoting internal balance. Spiritual wellness, the third pillar, encourages introspection, fostering inner peace and emotional resilience. In essence, embracing The Ruth Diet means embarking on a comprehensive journey towards healthier living, promoting a balance of body, mind, and spirit.

Let's explore these principles in detail.

Rejuvenation

Prepare to experience your body in an entirely new light. The Ruth Diet's rejuvenation aspect focuses on amplifying your body's innate healing abilities, helping you reclaim your youthful vitality and robust health. Through a unique blend of nutritional strategies and innovative wellness practices, the rejuvenation pillar invigorates you from within, promoting radiant skin, increased energy, and holistically improved well-being.

Detoxification

The Ruth Diet believes that a healthy body begins with a clean and balanced internal environment. The detoxification principle aims to free your body from toxins accumulated over time due to environmental exposure, poor dietary choices, and lifestyle habits. Harnessing the power of specific nutrient-dense foods and natural detoxification practices, the Diet aids you in flushing harmful substances from your body, facilitating healthier physiological operations, and rejuvenating your overall health.

Spiritual Wellness

The Ruth Diet doesn't neglect your spiritual health in pursuit of physical wellness. The spiritual wellness pillar recognises the profound connection between our mental, emotional, and spiritual states. It encourages practices that foster introspection, such as meditation, deep breathing, or even a simple stroll in nature. By nurturing inner peace and emotional resilience, the Ruth Diet helps you cultivate a balanced, serene mind that harmoniously complements your healthy body.

With the familiarity of these principles, you have only scratched the surface of what The Ruth Diet holds for you. As we delve deeper into subsequent chapters, you will unearth more profound aspects of this Diet that contribute to a full spectrum wellness experience.

So let us embark together on this transformative journey towards health, vitality, and a renewed spirit. Bid farewell to the conventional, one-sided approach to wellness, and embrace a comprehensive, all-encompassing pathway to health that The Ruth Diet offers. Ready to start your 30-day journey of rejuvenation? Here's to turning back the clock towards a newer, healthier you!

22

The Analogy of Ruth & The Transformational Lifestyle

Ruth, in biblical lore, was known for her indomitable spirit, unwavering faith, and remarkable transformation. Just like Ruth prepared to meet the king, we must gear up to embrace a transformative diet and lifestyle that manifests progress, rejuvenation, and holistic wellness.

As we embark on this journey, let us take a moment to immerse ourselves in the story of Ruth, which can be found in the Book of Ruth, a beautiful tale of love, loyalty, and divine providence. Reading this inspiring story will undoubtedly bolster our understanding of Ruth's transformation and illustrate a vivid backdrop against which the principles of The Ruth Diet can be explored.

Ruth's Preparation: An Analogy for Transformation

Ruth, a commoner by birth, underwent a significant metamorphosis in character and demeanor that transformed her into a revered figure, ultimately leading her to meet the king. Her journey stands as a paragon of growth, adaption, and remarkable transformation—a perfect analogy for our quest towards holistic wellness through The Ruth Diet.

As Ruth prepared herself to meet the king, she embraced various practices that honed her skills, purified her heart, and elevated her state of being. This journey mirrors our transformation as we incorporate elements of physical rejuvenation, spiritual wellness, and detoxification into our daily regimen.

Physical Rejuvenation

Like Ruth, we start by focusing on the physical body. Ruth prepared herself to meet the king by refining her physical appearance. In our case, we rejuvenate our bodies to meet a "kingly" state of optimum health and vitality. The recipes and exercises outlined in The Ruth Diet serve as our guidelines, empowering us to rejuvenate from within.

Detoxification

Ruth detoxified her life by eliminating adverse influences and experiences to transform herself. The Ruth Diet helps us detoxify by purging our bodies of accumulated toxins from poor diet choices, sedentary life habits, and environmental pollutants. Our detoxification journey lays the foundation for starting anew, much like Ruth.

Spiritual Wellness

Lastly, Ruth didn't just focus on her physical appearance; she also nurtured her spirit. She knew that her spiritual wellness was equally important in meeting the king. We, too, focus on nurturing our spirit, fostering peace, and cultivating emotional resilience. Through practices like meditation and mindfulness, we encourage our spiritual wellness, making it an integral part of The Ruth Diet.

The Transformational Lifestyle of The Ruth Diet

Following the Ruth analogy, The Ruth Diet is designed as a pathway to transformation. In embracing The Ruth Diet, we commit to grooming ourselves physically, cleansing our beings, and growing spiritually, just as Ruth did. This lifestyle embraces the thought that optimum health and vitality are achieved when there's a perfect balance of physical wellness, toxicity-free environment, and spiritual growth.

The Ruth Diet encourages us to view our journey towards wellness as an exciting chapter of transformation rather than a tedious task. Remember, Ruth's transformation was a journey, not an overnight event. This Diet isn't about short-term results, but about inculcating and embracing lifestyle changes that bring about sustained improvement.

As we progress along, much like Ruth's transformative journey, we'll learn more about The Ruth Diet's principles and how they can transform our lives, paving the way for a brighter, healthier future. After all, every king and queen deserves the finest preparations!

23

What to Expect from The Ruth Diet

Welcome to an exciting journey with The Ruth Diet, a transformative lifestyle modeled after the biblical character Ruth's incredible journey. This chapter unveils what to expect as you begin this voyage to holistic wellness, rejuvenation, and detoxification.

The Ruth Diet encourages you to rebalance your life, similar to the way Ruth redefined her path through purifying practices, physical refinement, and spiritual cultivation. It is a comprehensive approach to wellbeing that extends beyond mere dietary changes to encapsulate a broader spectrum of life's elements.

Dietary Rejuvenation through a 100% Liquid Diet

Imagine a rejuvenating diet filled with nourishing, liquid-based foods that support your body's optimal functionality. The Liquid Ruth Diet introduces you to an array of wholesome and nutrient-dense liquid foods that invigorate you from within. Say goodbye to fast food and processed snacks; it's time to relish liquid-based whole grains, fruits, vegetables, lean proteins, and healthy fats. With recipes catering to varied taste buds, you can expect to enjoy and benefit from numerous nutritious liquid meals.

Wholesome Liquid-Based Whole Grain Recipes

Incorporating whole grains into a liquid diet is a breeze with the Liquid Ruth Diet. We recommend nourishing and fiber-rich liquid-based recipes using whole grains such as oats, quinoa, and barley. Smoothies and blended porridges are perfect examples of ways to consume whole grains in liquid form while also packing a punch of nutrients. In this chapter, we will explore some delicious recipes that feature liquid-based whole grains that you can enjoy as part of the Liquid Ruth Diet.

Recipe 1: Hearty Oatmeal Smoothie

Ingredients:

- 1 cup almond milk
- 1/2 cup rolled oats, soaked in water for at least 30 minutes
- 1 ripe banana
- 1/4 cup plain Greek yogurt
- 1 tablespoon almond or peanut butter
- 1 tablespoon chia seeds
- 1/2 teaspoon ground cinnamon
- Optional: 1/2 cup ice

Instructions:

1. Blend all ingredients in a high-speed blender until smooth and creamy.
2. Adjust the consistency by adding more almond milk if desired.
3. Pour into a glass and enjoy immediately.

Recipe 2: Quinoa Breakfast Pudding

Ingredients:

- 1/2 cup cooked quinoa
- 1/2 cup almond milk
- 1/4 cup plain Greek yogurt
- 1 tablespoon honey or maple syrup
- 1/4 teaspoon vanilla extract
- 1/2 cup mixed berries

Instructions:

1. In a blender, combine cooked quinoa, almond milk, Greek yogurt, honey, and vanilla extract.
2. Blend on high speed until smooth and creamy.
3. Pour the pudding into a bowl and top with mixed berries.
4. Alternatively, you can create a layered parfait by alternating layers of quinoa pudding and berries in a tall glass.

Recipe 3: Barley and Vegetable Soup

Ingredients:

- 1 tablespoon olive oil
- 1 onion, chopped
- 2 cloves garlic, minced
- 1/2 cup barley, rinsed and drained
- 4 cups vegetable broth
- 1 cup diced carrots
- 1 cup diced celery
- 1 cup diced zucchini
- 1 teaspoon dried thyme

- Salt and pepper, to taste

Instructions:

1. Heat olive oil in a large pot. Add the onion and garlic and cook until soft and fragrant.
2. Add the barley and cook for a few minutes. Pour in the vegetable broth and bring to a boil.
3. Reduce heat and simmer for about 30 minutes, or until barley is tender.
4. Blend approx. 3/4 of the mixture in a blender until smooth (allow it to cool slightly before blending).
5. Pour the blended mixture back into the pot with the remaining un-blended soup.
6. Add the diced vegetables to the pot, along with the thyme, salt, and pepper.
7. Simmer for an additional 15-20 minutes, or until vegetables are tender.
8. Serve hot and enjoy!

These wholesome and delicious recipes showcase the potential of incorporating liquid-based whole grains into your diet. Enjoy the nutritious benefits of whole grains with these easy-to-make, flavorful creations that perfectly align with the principles of the Liquid Ruth Diet.

Nourishing Liquid Fruit and Vegetable Recipes

Embrace the bright colors and vibrant flavors of fruits and vegetables through the Liquid Ruth Diet. Our diet offers an array of ways to consume your daily servings of fruits and vegetables in a liquid form. From tantalizing smoothies and fresh juices to hearty pureed soups, here are some recipes to help you meet your daily fruit and vegetable intake.

Recipe 1: Green Power Smoothie

Ingredients:

- 1 cup spinach
- 1 ripe banana
- 1/2 cup sliced pineapple
- 1 tablespoon chia seeds
- 1 cup unsweetened almond milk

Instructions:

1. Place all the ingredients in a blender and blend until smooth.
2. Pour into a glass and enjoy immediately.

Recipe 2: Rainbow Carrot Juice

Ingredients:

- 5 rainbow carrots
- 2 apples
- 1/4 lemon, peeled
- 1 inch ginger root

Instructions:

1. Process all the ingredients through a juicer.
2. Stir the juice well before drinking.

Recipe 3: Refreshing Gazpacho Soup

Ingredients:

- 4 ripe tomatoes
- 1 cucumber, peeled and chopped
- 1 bell pepper, seeded and chopped
- 2 cloves garlic, peeled
- 1/4 cup olive oil
- 2 tablespoons vinegar
- Salt and pepper to taste

Instructions:

1. Blend all the ingredients in a blender or food processor until smooth.
2. Chill the soup in the refrigerator for at least 2 hours before serving.

These delightful liquid-based fruit and vegetable recipes serve as a simple and delicious way to fulfill your daily intake requirements. Experiment with these recipes and discover the enjoyment and health benefits that come alongside the Liquid Ruth Diet.

Delectable Liquid Lean Protein Recipes

Amplify your protein intake with the Liquid Ruth Diet's impressive selection of protein-rich, liquid-based recipes. These nourishing smoothies, satisfying cold soups, and nutrient-dense beverages supply you with lean proteins that contribute to muscle development and bolster your immune system. Here are some recipe examples to incorporate into your diet.

Recipe 1: Vanilla-Banana Protein Smoothie

Ingredients:

- 1 ripe banana
- 1 cup unsweetened almond milk
- 1 scoop vanilla protein powder
- 1 tablespoon almond butter
- A handful of ice cubes

Instructions:

1. Place all ingredients into a high-speed blender.
2. Blend until smooth and frothy.
3. Pour into a glass and enjoy immediately.

Recipe 2: Cold Lentil and Tahini Soup

Ingredients:

- 1 cup cooked red lentils
- 1 garlic clove
- 1 tablespoon tahini
- 1 tablespoon olive oil
- Salt and pepper to taste
- Lemon juice from half a lemon
- 2 cups water or vegetable broth

Instructions:

1. Combine all ingredients in a blender.
2. Blend until smooth.
3. Chill in the refrigerator before serving.

Recipe 3: Almond-Protein Shake

Ingredients:

- 1 cup unsweetened almond milk
- 1 scoop chocolate protein powder
- 1 tablespoon almond butter
- 1 tablespoon cocoa powder
- A handful of ice cubes

Instructions:

1. In a blender, combine all ingredients.
2. Blend until smooth.
3. Pour into a glass and enjoy.

These protein-rich recipes bring dynamic flavors and beneficial nutrients to your daily diet. Through the Liquid Ruth Diet, you can enjoy innovative ways of consuming lean proteins and enrich your overall health.

Luscious Liquid Healthy Fat Recipes

The Liquid Ruth Diet ensures your body receives vital healthy fats needed to support brain function, immune health, and overall well-being. By integrating high-quality fat sources such as avocados, nut and seed butters, and cold-pressed oils, the diet presents a variety of mouthwatering smoothies, soups, and liquid-based recipes.

Recipe 1: Creamy Avocado Smoothie

Ingredients:

- 1 ripe avocado, pitted and peeled
- 1 ripe banana

- 1 cup unsweetened almond milk
- 1 tablespoon honey or maple syrup
- 1/2 teaspoon vanilla extract
- A handful of ice cubes

Instructions:

1. Place all ingredients into a high-speed blender.
2. Blend until silky smooth.
3. Pour into a glass and enjoy immediately.

Recipe 2: Nutty Carrot Soup

Ingredients:

- 2 cups chopped carrots
- 1 cup water or vegetable broth
- 1/4 cup almond butter
- 1 tablespoon cold-pressed coconut oil
- Salt and pepper, to taste
- 1 teaspoon ground cinnamon

Instructions:

1. Steam the carrots until tender.
2. Place cooked carrots, water or vegetable broth, almond butter, coconut oil, salt, pepper, and cinnamon into a blender.
3. Blend until smooth and creamy.
4. Serve warm or chilled, as preferred.

Recipe 3: Seed Butter Shake

Ingredients:

- 1 cup unsweetened almond milk
- 1 banana, sliced and frozen
- 2 tablespoons pumpkin seed butter (or substitute with sunflower seed butter)
- 1 teaspoon chia seeds
- 1 teaspoon flaxseeds
- A dash of cinnamon
- A handful of ice cubes

Instructions:

1. Combine all ingredients in a blender.
2. Blend until smooth and frosty.
3. Pour into a glass and enjoy.

Embrace the benefits of these diverse and scrumptious liquid healthy fat recipes. The Liquid Ruth Diet provides new and exciting ways to incorporate essential nutrients into your daily meals and enhance your overall health.

Liquid Diet Recipes for Varied Taste Buds

The Liquid Ruth Diet offers a multitude of scrumptious recipes that appeal to diverse tastes. The diet includes flavors from around the world, with different combinations of fruits, vegetables, nuts, seeds, and whole grains. You'll find satisfying savory soups, tropical smoothies, and everything in between.

In conclusion, the Liquid Ruth Diet delivers revitalizing properties through its comprehensive approach, utilizing 100% liquid-based meals that promote optimal bodily function and overall wellness.

Maintaining a liquid diet doesn't have to be monotonous or bland; explore the world of nutrient-dense, liquid-based foods and experience the rejuvenation the Liquid Ruth Diet has to offer.

Physical & Environmental Detoxification

Detoxification is more than a cleanse; it's a renewing process that removes harmful toxins from our bodies and our surroundings. To embody Ruth's transformation, The Ruth Diet will guide you through dietary detoxification strategies that eliminate toxins resulting from pre-existing poor dietary habits. It will also offer practical tips to detoxify your environment, thereby reducing the exposure to external pollutants, which is as equally essential as internal cleansing.

Spiritual Wellbeing

Mental and spiritual wellbeing hold a significant place in the Ruth Diet. Ruth's transformation was steered by her robust spirit and mental resilience, and we model our journey similarly. On this path, you'll be exposed to practices that help cultivate inner peace, clarity, and emotional resilience. Mindfulness techniques, breathing exercises, outdoor activities, and periods of silent reflection are some of the aspects we'll explore.

Endurance and Anticipating Results

Just as Ruth's transformation wasn't overnight, you shouldn't expect immediate results from The Ruth Diet. This diet is about embracing a sustainable lifestyle change for long-term wellness and vitality. Significant transformations take time, and you're advised to exhibit patience and stick with the guidelines. The Ruth Diet emphasizes developing enduring habits that lead to sustained wellness, not temporary quick fixes.

Support and Guidance

As you navigate The Ruth Diet, expect consistent support and guidance to make this journey as smooth as possible. E-books, newsletters, updates and Q&A sessions are all part of The Ruth Diet's structure. Our aim is to provide you with all the resources and motivation needed to embrace this transformative lifestyle successfully.

By choosing The Ruth Diet, you're deciding to better yourself on multiple fronts – physically, environmentally, and spiritually. Just as Ruth did centuries ago, you have decided to change the course of your life – to become healthier, happier, and more balanced. And remember, just like Ruth, this transformation is a journey, not a destination. So, embrace the journey, learn, grow, and reach for your "kingly" state of wellbeing.

VIII

Advancing with Science: The Backbone of The Ruth Diet

24

Advancing with Science: The Backbone of The Ruth Diet

Welcome to the realm where science meets The Ruth Diet. This chapter unravels the scientific underpinnings behind the concept of "turning back time"—an analogy for rejuvenation, renewal, and the remarkable transformations possible with The Ruth Diet.

Rejuvenation and The Science Behind It

Every aspect of The Ruth Diet is rooted in scientific evidence. From nutritional plans to the suggested physical activities, everything is designed based on scientific research in health, nutrition, and wellness.

Rejuvenation, a core principle of The Ruth Diet, leans on a biological phenomenon of cellular renewal. Many of our body's cells are continually replicating and replacing older cells. This aspect of human physiology allows us to recover from injuries and illnesses. By following the rejuvenation principles of The Ruth Diet, we can optimally bolster this process for increased vitality.

Detoxification: Scientific Rationale

Environmental and dietary toxins can accumulate in our bodies, affecting our health and wellness. The detoxifying aspect of The Ruth Diet is to mitigate the impact of these toxins. Scientific research highlights that a diet filled with certain types of foods (rich in antioxidants, for example) can aid in the elimination of toxins from our bodies. Furthermore, detoxifying our environment, like improving air quality, reducing noise pollution, and using chemical-free household products, can significantly impact our overall health and well-being.

Spiritual Wellness from a Scientific Perspective

The spiritual component of The Ruth Diet might seem to lie outside the scientific domain, but many scientific studies support the positive impact of mindfulness, meditation, and other spiritual practices on health. They can reduce stress, enhance mental clarity, improve emotional stability, and contribute to overall well-being. Hence, cultivating spiritual wellness fits neatly within the scientific approach to holistic health that The Ruth Diet embodies.

Taking a Longer-Term View: Inculcating Sustainable Habits

Remember, the transformation The Ruth Diet promises isn't overnight but incremental. Psychological science supports the notion that building sustainable habits takes time. As we progress through The Ruth Diet, we will gradually curb unhealthy practices and replace them with healthy ones, in alignment with scientific strategies for habit formation.

Trusting the Science

In essence, the entire framework of The Ruth Diet stands tall on a scientific foundation, making it a substantial and reliable pathway for health and wellness transformation. As you move ahead and begin to experience the benefits, let scientific reasoning be your reassuring guide. Rest assured, every aspect of The Ruth Diet—from dietary changes to enhancing spirituality—is rooted in science, advancing you towards holistic wellness.

25

Benefits of a 30-day commitment each year to The Ruth Die

A consistent and deliberate practice of self-care, rejuvenation, and self-improvement has a profound impact on our lives, and establishing a 30-day commitment each year to The Ruth Diet is a monumental step towards embracing a holistic lifestyle transformation. This chapter reveals the myriad benefits of dedicating 30 days of each year to experiencing the refreshing and revitalizing effects of The Ruth Diet on your body, mind, and spirit.

1. Establishing and Strengthening Habits

Taking part in a 30-day commitment to The Ruth Diet each year serves as an opportunity to establish and reinforce healthy habits.It allows you to dive further into the practices and teachings brought forth by The Ruth Diet while providing a framework for building and maintaining better choices in nutrition, exercise, and spiritual development.

2. Renewed Focus on Holistic Health

Life tends to throw countless distractions and challenges our way, steering us away from the path of holistic wellness. Dedicating 30 days each year to focus on The Ruth Diet helps you regain that focus, reconnecting you with the process of rejuvenation, detoxification, and spiritual growth.

3. Deepened Spiritual Connection

Your 30-day commitment serves as a yearly period of reflection, providing an opportunity to deepen your spiritual connection. Through practices like meditation, mindfulness, and even acts of kindness or gratitude, you can solidify your spiritual roots during this dedicated time.

4. Assessing Progress and Adjusting Goals

A yearly 30-day evaluation period allows you to assess your progress and achievements and make any necessary adjustments to your goals, ensuring they align with your current needs and aspirations. This periodic review helps to keep you on track, motivated, and committed to your health journey.

5. Enhanced Energy and Vitality

Focusing on The Ruth Diet for 30 days a year ensures that your body, mind, and spirit receive a concentrated dose of revitalization. This boosts your energy levels and vitality, making you feel more alive and in alignment with your optimal health.

6. Encouragement for Long-term Success

By committing to a 30-day period of focus each year, you prioritize your health and wellbeing even as life's demands evolve. This dedication sets off a ripple effect that encourages you to maintain the lifestyle changes throughout the year, leading to long-term success in maintaining a healthy, balanced life.

In conclusion, a 30-day commitment to The Ruth Diet can create a powerful yearly tradition, manifesting in significant physical, mental, and spiritual benefits that echo throughout the year. By dedicating this time, you're actively prioritizing your well-being while setting yourself up for success in the long run.

26

Latest research and supportive evidence

As we continue our journey with The Ruth Diet, our comprehensive exploration of the most recent scientific literature reaffirms the principles and practices inherent in this transformative lifestyle. Backed by its robust scientific foundation, this enhanced chapter aims to give you deeper insights into the science and studies that form the foundation of The Ruth Diet.

Expanded View on Nutritional Principles

Emerging research converges on the wisdom that underscores the nutritional principles championed by The Ruth Diet. A multitude of recent studies emphasize the benefits derived from the consumption of a balanced diet comprising whole foods such as fruits, vegetables, lean proteins, and healthy fats. This includes a wide array of research showing that incorporating such a dietary approach protects against various chronic diseases, helps improve mental health, enhances overall health, and contributes significantly to longer life span.

Detailed Insights into Detoxification and Environmental Health

In this era of increasing environmental challenges, research continues to establish an undeniable link between environmental health and personal well-being. A cache of current studies conclusively finds that reducing exposure to environmental toxins—both airborne and those embedded in our day-to-day items—can significantly decrease the risk of a plethora of health conditions. The Ruth Diet's advocacy for cleansing the body and sanitizing our surroundings holds an elevated level of importance in this environmentally compromised time.

Comprehensive Perspective on Physical Activity and Wellness

The importance of physical activity in promoting overall health is undeniable. Still, recent research goes a step further by highlighting its role in domains beyond just physical fitness. Newer studies emphasize the role exercise plays in mental wellness, cognitive functioning, and even enhancing longevity. By choosing to incorporate regular exercise, as The Ruth Diet encourages, you will find yourself on the path toward comprehensive wellness.

Deepened Understanding of Spiritual Practices for Overall Health

More than ever, modern researchers are keen on exploring the science behind spiritual practices like meditation and mindfulness. A barrage of studies now supports the contention that these practices can help manage stress, boost mood, improve life quality, and even foster better body-mind connectivity. As The Ruth Diet guides you towards these practices, you can find comfort in the array of scientific evidence supporting their benefits on mental and emotional health.

Better Appreciation of Sustainable Habit Building

Instead of fostering short-term fixes, The Ruth Diet strongly advocates for long-term, sustainable lifestyle changes. A panoply of research echoes this stance, demonstrating how enduring changes lead to enhanced morale, reduced risk of disease, and an overall better lifestyle satisfaction.

In conclusion, the approach of The Ruth Diet aligns effortlessly with the multitude of recent research findings spanning nutrition, detoxification, physical activity, spiritual practices, and habit formation. This continuous corroboration from the scientific community and field experts further solidifies the Diet's foundations, making it a compelling and trustworthy model for holistic health and well-being enhancement.

IX

Revealing the Physical Health Benefits of The Ruth Diet

27

Revealing the Physical Health Benefits of The Ruth Diet

As we journey further into The Ruth Diet, this chapter presents a comprehensive focus on the myriad physical health benefits derived from this lifestyle. Let's dive into a detailed examination on the substantial influence of The Ruth Diet on physical health, underpinned by cutting-edge scientific research and everyday experiences.

Extensive Benefits on Nutritional Health

By advocating a balanced, portion-controlled diet abundant in whole, nutrient-dense foods, The Ruth Diet drastically improves nutritional health. Regular consumption of an assortment of fruits, vegetables, lean proteins, and healthy fats ensures a well-rounded intake of essential nutrients. This diverse nutrient profile fuels optimal bodily function, reinforces the immune system, and cultivates overall vitality, laying the foundation for a healthier you.

Astounding Improvements on Digestive Health

The Ruth Diet offers excellent solutions for improved digestive health. With recommendations rooted in regular detoxification, sufficient hydration, and fiber-rich diet, it fosters a harmonious gut environment. This regime supports gut-cleansing, promotes the growth of beneficial flora, enhances nutrient absorption, and combats digestive distress. As a result, a balanced gut contributes to overall well-being and disease resistance.

Powerful Strengthening of Cardiovascular Health

The regimen of regular physical activity and a diet low in saturated fats but populated with heart-healthy foods forms the core of The Ruth Diet's enhancement of cardiovascular health. Besides, the advocacy for stress management techniques aids in heart health. This multifaceted approach helps moderate blood pressure, maintain healthy cholesterol levels, and mitigate the risk of cardiovascular diseases, underlining the significance of heart health in general well-being.

Notable Boost in Metabolic Health

Integration of The Ruth Diet alters the metabolic paradigm for the better. It elevates the metabolic rate and fosters balanced blood sugar levels through a purposeful combination of regular exercise and a balanced diet brimming with all essential macro and micronutrients. It paves the way for effective weight management and can dramatically lower the risk of metabolic syndrome and related disorders.

Optimization of Bone and Joint Health

With a strategic focus on weight-bearing exercises supplemented with a diet rich in bone-nurturing nutrients like calcium, vitamin D, and magnesium, The Ruth Diet is instrumental in preserving bone density and joint agility.

It presents a substantial preventive measure against conditions such as osteoporosis, arthritis, and other movement-related ailments, ensuring mobility and flexibility as you age.

Remarkable Enhancement in Skin Health

The Ruth Diet forges a path to radiant skin health. Through mindful practices like sufficient hydration, the consumption of antioxidant-rich foods, and regular detoxification, it contributes to maintaining skin's elasticity, combating early signs of aging, and fostering a healthy glow. The skin, being the largest organ and a mirror reflecting internal health, reaps visible benefits from these practices.

In summary, the profound impact of The Ruth Diet on physical health spans an extensive spectrum, addressing crucial aspects from heart health and digestive wellness to metabolic balance, bone strength, and skin health. It holistically elevates physical health, laying a robust foundation for a vibrant and energetic life, embodying the transformational power of this lifestyle.

28

Concentrated Focus on Skin Rejuvenation and Overall Health Transformation

In this all-encompassing chapter, we delve into the influential role The Ruth Diet plays in skin rejuvenation and the interconnectedness of skin health with overall well-being. Discover how this nurturing lifestyle's recommendations contribute to promoting a youthful appearance and boosting overall health at the same time.

Skin Rejuvenation through Nutrient Infusion

The Ruth Diet accentuates the importance of consuming essential nutrients for skin health. Its principles prioritize the intake of vitamins A, C, and E, as well as zinc, selenium, and omega-3 fatty acids, which contribute to rejuvenating the skin, reducing inflammation, and enhancing elasticity.

Cellular Renewal and Detoxification

By promoting regular detoxification and sufficient hydration, The Ruth Diet helps flush out toxins from the body. This practice empowers cellular renewal, supports collagen production, and aids in maintaining skin's elasticity, all vital factors for skin rejuvenation.

The Power of Antioxidants

The Ruth Diet encourages the consumption of antioxidant-rich foods, such as berries, leafy greens, and nuts. These antioxidants actively combat harmful free radicals, minimizing oxidative stress, and helping to prevent premature aging.

Sun Protection and Skincare Routine

The Ruth Diet recognizes the significance of implementing a strategic skincare routine that includes sun protection. This practice safeguards the skin against harmful UV rays and prevents sun damage, contributing to a youthful, radiant appearance.

Holistic Health and Skin Restoration

At its core, The Ruth Diet is a holistic approach to overall health and wellness. By emphasizing mental and emotional well-being, exercise, nutrition, and detoxification, it fosters healthier body systems that reflect positively on skin health.

In conclusion, The Ruth Diet offers a comprehensive approach to skin rejuvenation and overall health transformation. By adhering to this nurturing lifestyle, not only will you be working towards revitalizing your skin for a more youthful look, but also committing to an all-encompassing journey of internal health, wellness, and vitality.

29

Exploring the Power of the Body's Natural Healing and the Role of Diet

In this enlightening chapter, we delve into the captivating realm of the body's natural healing prowess and the paramount role diet plays in this process. Discover the fascinating mechanisms behind the body's self-healing capabilities, and how following The Ruth Diet can empower this innate process.

Unraveling the Body's Natural Healing Process

At its core, the human body has an incredible capability to heal and repair itself. This natural healing process involves intricate cellular repair mechanisms, immune system responses, and hormonal regulation. The body's innate healing power can address both minor injuries like skin cuts as well as chronic conditions, given the right support and adequate time.

Role of Diet in Healing

Diet plays a vital role in supporting the body's natural healing process. Nutrient-rich foods provide the necessary building blocks required by the body to repair damaged tissues, combat infections, and maintain the optimal functioning of the immune system. The Ruth Diet, with its emphasis on nutrient-dense, whole foods, delivers the necessary nourishment the body needs to facilitate the healing process.

Diet that Fosters Immune Function

The Ruth Diet encourages the consumption of foods rich in antioxidants, omega-3 fatty acids, vitamins, and minerals, all of which are crucial for robust immune system function. A strong immune system enhances the body's defense mechanism against illnesses and optimizes the natural healing process.

Probiotics and Gut Health in Immunity

The Ruth Diet also advocates the incorporation of probiotics into one's daily nutritional plan. Probiotics, which are beneficial bacteria typically present in fermented foods like yogurt, sauerkraut, and kimchi, help maintain a healthy gut environment. This is significant because gut health is closely tied to immune function, and a well-balanced gut microbiome bolsters the body's natural defenses.

Nutrition for Cellular Repair and Regeneration

The Ruth Diet emphasizes the intake of lean proteins, essential fatty acids, and a variety of fruits and vegetables, all of which contribute to cellular repair and regeneration. These foods provide the nutrients necessary to promote cellular health, aiding in the body's self-healing mechanisms.

Hydration and Healing

Adequate hydration is an often overlooked but crucial component of the healing process. The Ruth Diet stresses the importance of drinking sufficient water throughout the day, as it helps transport nutrients and oxygen to cells, aids in toxin removal, and keeps tissues healthy and pliable.

Diet and Hormonal Balance

Hormonal imbalances can impede the body's ability to heal and function optimally. The Ruth Diet adopts a holistic approach to health, focusing on foods and lifestyle practices that support hormonal balance. Proper balance of hormones facilitates optimal healing and overall health.

Stress Management and Healing

Stress can negatively impact hormone levels and hinder the body's healing process. Thus, The Ruth Diet promotes stress management techniques, such as meditation, yoga, and regular exercise, to curtail the adverse effects of stress on hormonal balance and healing.

In conclusion, the comprehensive approach of The Ruth Diet readily supports the body's natural healing process, endorsing robust immune function, efficient cellular repair, and hormonal balance. Embracing this enriching lifestyle can significantly bolster your body's innate healing capabilities, promoting overall wellness and vitality.

X

Power of Detox: Teas and Liquid Silver

30

The Power of Detox Teas and Liquid Silver During Your Liquid Fast

The Liquid Ruth Diet extends beyond merely abstaining from solid food. It incorporates detox teas and liquid silver, creating a potent combination to support your regimen, cleanse your body, and uplift your spirit.

Detox teas form the cornerstone of the diet throughout the early hours. These herbal tonic infusions bring together a symphony of carefully selected ingredients rich in antioxidants and anti-inflammatory properties, kick-starting your body's cleansing process each day.

- **Nettle Leaf Tea**: A powerhouse of vitamins and minerals, nettle leaf tea aids in the removal of metabolic wastes and promotes renal excretion due to diuretic properties; this helps detoxify and purify the body.
- **Dandelion Root Tea**: A known detoxifier, dandelion root tea supports the liver, aiding digestion and spurring the body's natural detoxification processes.
- **Burdock Tea**: This root tea contains compounds known to purge toxins from the bloodstream, promoting skin health and contributing to overall body detoxification.

These potent herbs stimulate the liver, enhance digestion, and support the body's detoxification processes, all while their refreshing flavors provide a rejuvenating start to your day.

As your day progresses, the incorporation of **liquid silver** makes its appearance. A highly underestimated elixir, colloidal silver has been suggested to possess powerful antimicrobial potential. Employed judiciously within the Ruth Diet, it aids in maintaining gut health, potentially working to balance the intestinal flora while keeping potential infections at bay. This ensures that the cleansing process undergoes smoothly, with minimal interruption due to any potential infections or imbalances.

Through the careful integration of detox teas and liquid silver in the Liquid Ruth diet, you embark on a holistic journey towards well-being. Coupled with mindfulness practices, these elements enable you to purify the body, renew your spirit, and steel you for the adventure ahead.

Experiment with different options and discover your favorite detox tea. The Ruth Diet's flexibility allows you to choose from various teas, each offering unique benefits, adding a personal touch to your wellness journey.

31

How to correctly use these components for maximum effect

In the journey of the Ruth Diet, the effective utilization of both detox teas and liquid silver is paramount. While their inclusion in the diet can facilitate a thorough detox and cleanse, it's key to understand how to correctly use these components for maximum effect.

The Art of Brewing Detox Teas

Brewing detox teas is more about precision than it is about complication. Here are a few simple steps on how to properly prepare your detox tea:

1. **Choosing the tea**: Opt for high-quality, organic tea leaves. In the Ruth Diet, nettle leaf, dandelion root, and burdock teas are premium choices known for their extensive detoxifying benefits.
2. **Steeping the tea**: A general rule of thumb is to steep your chosen tea for approximately 5-10 minutes in boiling water, infusing all the essential oils and beneficial compounds within the water.
3. **Frequency**: The beauty of these detox teas lies in their versatility. They can be relished morning, afternoon, or evening. However, note that it's recommended to start your day with a warm cup of detox tea for a

rejuvenating wake-up call to your system.

A Just measure of Liquid Silver

In the realm of liquid silver or colloidal silver, moderation is key. Here's how you can incorporate its goodness in your regime:

1. **Dosage**: Start small, with 3 teaspoon of silver in a day, and observe how your body responds to it. Gradually increase the dose to a maximum of one tablespoon per day, as per comfort and need.
2. **Timing**: Preference is typically to consume liquid silver in the latter half of the day, enabling its antimicrobial properties to work while you rest.
3. **Patterns of Consumption**: Liquid silver should be consumed in cycles, such as 10 days on, then 2 days off, to allow the body to effectively use the liquid without fostering dependency.

Remember, the Ruth Diet emphasizes balance above all. It's paramount to listen to your body and adjust the regimen as necessary, as every individual responds differently to detoxification processes. Equipped with these instructions, unlock the full potential of detox teas and liquid silver to turbocharge your detox journey and create an invigorating experience that suits your unique needs.

32

Common queries and their solutions

In this chapter, we address common questions related to the use of detox teas and liquid silver as vital components of the Liquid Ruth Diet, ensuring their optimum effectiveness.

Detox Teas

Q1: Can I drink detox teas cold or is it necessary to have them hot?

The potency of detox teas does not vary significantly between cold and hot states. Therefore, you can enjoy them as per your preference. However, as the main goal is to stimulate detoxification, a warm cup of tea can have a soothing effect and enhance hydration.

Q2: Is there any disadvantage if I steep the tea for less than 5 minutes or more than 10 minutes?

The steeping time influences the extraction of beneficial compounds from the tea leaves into the water. If the steeping time is too short, the tea may not release all beneficial components. On the other hand, steeping it for too long might lead to a stronger infusion which could alter the taste and potentially strain the digestive system.

Liquid Silver

Q3: What will happen if I consume more than the recommended dosage of liquid silver?

It's advisable to start small and listen to your body. Too much liquid silver might upset your gut balance as it could disrupt both harmful and beneficial bacteria. Always stick to the recommended dosage and cycle pattern for safe and effective detox.

Q4: Can I mix liquid silver with other liquids?

Yes, you can mix liquid silver with water or juice. However, avoid mixing it with salty solutions, chlorine, or any protein-based liquids as it could potentially reduce its effectiveness.

General

Q5: Can I continue to take my regular medications while on this detox regimen?

Before starting any new diet or detox regimen, including the Liquid Ruth Diet, it's of the utmost importance to consult with your healthcare provider, especially if you are currently taking any medications.

Navigating through any new regimen might seem overwhelming, but armed with the right knowledge and guidance, you are all set to embark on this transformative detox journey. Remember, consistency is key, patience is a virtue, and your health is your wealth.

XI

Daily Facials & Extensive Skincare Routine: Emphasis on Skin Health

33

The Importance of Skin Health in the Overall Wellness Journey

An all-encompassing approach to wellness is incomplete without adequate attention to skin health. As our body's largest organ, the skin acts as both a barrier and a channel for exchange between the inside and the outside world. Therefore, maintaining skin health holistically amplifies the overall wellness journey.

The Many Roles of Skin

Understanding the skin's functions highlights why its health is indispensable to our overall well-being:

1. **Protection**: Our skin acts as a shield, guarding against environmental hazards, pathogens, and physical injuries.
2. **Temperature regulation**: Through varying blood flow and the process of sweating, the skin helps maintain body temperature.
3. **Sensory perception**: Rich in sensory receptors, the skin allows us to experience touch, temperature, pressure, and pain.
4. **Excretion**: By eliminating sweat and oils, the skin aids in the expulsion of waste and toxins.

The Skin-Wellness Connection

Harmonizing skin health bolsters general well-being in myriad ways:

- **Stress relief**: A skincare routine that includes relaxing techniques like facial massages or warm detox baths can lower stress and anxiety levels.
- **Quality sleep**: Diminishing skin issues such as itching or discomfort can lead to better sleep quality, promoting overall wellness.
- **Boosting self-esteem**: Radiant, healthy skin enhances one's appearance, bolstering confidence and self-assurance.
- **Immune system support**: Ensuring skin integrity helps prevent infections and supports the body's immune responses.

Developing a Holistic Approach

To nurture skin health as part of your wellness journey, consider the following:

- **Diet**: Consume a balanced diet, abundant in antioxidants, healthy fats, and vitamins, to nourish your skin from within.
- **Hydration**: Adequate water intake helps maintain skin elasticity, aids in detoxification, and supports essential bodily functions.
- **Exercise**: Engaging in physical activity boosts blood flow, supplying the skin with oxygen and nutrients, while promoting toxin elimination through sweat.
- **Natural skincare**: Choosing natural products and ingredients for your skincare routine can help reduce exposure to harmful chemicals while supporting skin health.

Embracing the interdependence of skin health and general well-being is integral to a truly holistic wellness journey. Nurturing and cherishing our skin reciprocates the love and attentiveness we invest in it, allowing us to feel our best both inside and out.

<h1 style="text-align:center">34</h1>

Practical Guidance on Daily Facials for Refreshed Skin

Embracing skincare as an integral part of wellness doesn't have to be complicated; a few dedicated minutes in your daily routine can contribute to preserving the vitality of your skin. Designed to cleanse, restore, and beautify, daily facials offer an ideal regimen towards imbuing skin health.

My Personal Regimen

To give a glimpse into my approach, my personal regimen includes a Facial Mask, Turmeric Facial Soap, Turmeric, Rosewater, Rosehip, Lavender Toner, and Turmeric and Rosehip Plant–Based Facial Creme.

Personalizing Your Regimen

For effective facial care, it's paramount to tune into your skin's particular requirements. Recognize your skin's type and needs while also accounting for lifestyle and environmental factors.

Building a Basic Routine

A daily facial routine typically comprises three essential steps—cleansing, toning, and moisturizing.

- **Cleansing**: Initiate your routine with a gentle cleanser, eliminating the day's grime and preparing your skin for further treatment. The Turmeric Facial Soap from The Apothecary Farmacy can be a fitting start, combining cleansing efficacy with the nurturing attributes of turmeric.
- **Toning**: Next, toning clears remaining residuals, tightens pores, and rebalances the skin's pH. Try the plant-infused Turmeric Toner from The Apothecary Farmacy for a soothing refreshment.
- **Moisturizing**: Conclude the routine with a hydrating moisturizer. A plant-based turmeric facial cream will not only hydrate the skin but also incorporate the anti-inflammatory and antioxidant benefits of turmeric.

Including Optional Add-Ons

Beyond the basics, you can personalize and enrich your routine with treatments targeting specific skin issues or for additional nourishment.

- **Exfoliating**: Regular gentle exfoliation, using a scrub or a mask like the Turmeric 3 Clay blend, can clear away dead skin cells and instigate a vibrant complexion.
- **Serums and oils**: These concentrated potions can address specific skin conditions or provide added hydration.
- **Facial massages**: Integrating facial massages can stimulate blood flow, support lymphatic drainage, and promote a relaxed glow.

Consistency is Key

Remember, consistent care yields the most beneficial results. Despite its simplicity, sticking to a basic daily routine will work wonders in maintaining your skin's health and resilience.

Living the Message

By advocating daily facials, the aim is not to accomplish perfection but to foster an appreciation for the skin you're in. Engaging in this active self-care ritual is a celebration of your unique beauty, and a testament to your commitment to overall wellness.

35

Comprehensive, Step-by-Step Skincare Routine to Promote Youthful Skin

A well-organized skincare routine is more than just a beauty regimen; it's a testament to one's overall wellness. Emphasizing skin health translates to an engaged commitment in caring for ourselves, propelling us toward achieving a youthful glow that mirrors our inner vitality.

Preliminary Step: Understanding Your Skin

Before embarking on the journey of skincare, understanding your skin type is essential. It enables a tailored skincare routine that caters specifically to your skin's requirements.

Step 1: Cleansing

The initial step is cleansing, a critical practice to whisk away accumulated dirt, oil, and makeup. Employing a gentle cleanser such as Turmeric Facial Soap ensures skin isn't stripped of its natural oils.

Step 2: Toning

Follow the cleansing action with a toner to remove any residual cleanser, rebalance the skin's pH, and prepare your skin for subsequent products. An ideal choice would be a plant-infused turmeric toner, providing soothing hydration and balance.

Step 3: Exfoliation

While not an everyday step, exfoliating once or twice a week can help remove dead skin cells, revealing a fresh, bright complexion. Remember to employ gentle methods like a scrub or a mask, such as the Turmeric 3 Clay blend.

Step 4: Serum and Oil Application

Serums and oils are concentrated treatments targeting specific skin concerns or providing added hydration. Following the exfoliation, apply your chosen product to an already clean and receptive face for maximum skin benefits.

Step 5: Moisturizing

The subsequent phase is moisturizing. Flatly not to neglect this step; even oily skin needs moisturization. Try the plant-based Turmeric and Rosehip Facial Cream for an enriched, hydrating experience.

Step 6: Sun Protection

Last but never least, sun protection is crucial. Sun damage contributes significantly to premature skin aging. Therefore, always don a broad-spectrum sunblock, even during cloudy days.

Final Thoughts

Patience is vital as results don't emerge overnight. Your commitment to yourself, consistency, and gusto will culminate in the ultimate reward—healthy, youthful skin.

XII

Hydrate and Detoxify: Drinking Water and Castor Oil Packs

36

Hydrate and Detoxify: Drinking Water and Castor Oil Packs

In the journey towards holistic wellness during The Ruth Diet, hydration assumes a pivotal role. When the body is adequately hydrated, it functions optimally, promoting overall health. Additionally, the usage of Castor Oil packs lends a helping hand, fostering detoxification and contributing further to the wellness protocol.

Role of Hydration in The Ruth Diet

Hydration serves as a fundamental element in any diet, and The Ruth Diet is no exception. Regular, sufficient water intake aids digestion, facilitates the elimination of waste, and optimizes metabolic function, thereby strengthening the efficacy of the diet.

The Merits of Drinking Water

Water, the elixir of life even in its simplicity, offers several benefits, especially during a dietary regimen:

- **Enhances metabolism**: Adequate hydration fosters an efficient metabolic function, thereby promoting weight management.

- **Maintains balance**: Water is vital to maintaining the balance of bodily fluids, including digestion, absorption, circulation, and temperature regulation.
- **Boosts skin health**: Regular water intake aids in maintaining optimal skin hydration and supports detoxification, leading to healthier and clearer skin.

Introduction to Castor Oil Packs

As an ancient remedy, castor oil paves the way for a potent addition to your wellness routine. Castor oil packs—flannel cloths soaked in castor oil and applied to the skin—provide an effective way to reap the benefits of this healing oil.

Benefits of Castor Oil Packs

Castor oil packs provide their unique benefits:

- **Promotes detoxification**: Castor oil packs aid in the body's natural detoxification process, supporting liver function and aiding in the removal of toxins.
- **Anti-inflammatory benefits**: Castor oil has anti-inflammatory properties, making its packs beneficial in relieving pain, inflammation, and swelling.
- **Supports digestion**: Regular use of castor oil packs can improve digestion and alleviate constipation.

Conclusion: Integrating Hydration and Castor Oil Packs in The Ruth Diet

Incorporating sufficient hydration and the usage of castor oil packs in The Ruth Diet underscores a holistic approach to wellness, bolstering the diet's potency and benefiting the overall health and well-being.

37

Exploring the Usefulness of Castor Oil Packs for Detoxification

Inherent within traditional healing practices are remedies that stand the test of time, with castor oil packs being a quintessential example. Revered for their undeniable contributions towards detoxification and pain relief, castor oil packs have secured their rightful place within the wellness regime.

Understanding Castor Oil Packs

Castor oil packs involve the topical application of castor oil—typically through soaking a piece of flannel in the oil, applying it to the skin, and placing a heat source over it. The heat helps the oil penetrate deeply, thus amplifying its potential benefits.

Castor Oil and Detoxification

The detoxifying benefits of castor oil packs primarily root from their support towards liver function. With the liver being a primary organ in our body's detoxification process, the packs can aid in the removal of harmful toxins.

ThE Mechanism of Action

Castor oil packs exploit the anti-inflammatory and lymph-stimulating effects of castor oil. Here's how it works:

1. Heat application promotes absorption - The heat applied over the castor oil pack enhances skin permeability, letting the oil infiltrate into the body.
2. Stimulation of the lymphatic system - The absorbed oil stimulates the lymphatic system, promoting the body's natural detoxification mechanism.
3. Liver function support - Castor oil's properties help the liver operate more efficiently, thereby assisting in the clearance of toxins and waste products.

Potential Benefits of Castor Oil Packs for Detoxification

- **Supports the liver**: Castor oil packs provide ancillary support to the liver, aiding in the management of digestion and detoxification.
- **Promotes clear skin**: By assisting with detoxification, castor oil packs can help promote clear skin.
- **Aids digestion**: Regular use of castor oil packs can enhance the digestive system's health and potentially alleviate issues like constipation.

Efficient Use of Castor Oil Packs

For the most effective use of castor oil packs, place them over the liver and allow them to work for about one hour. Remember to rest while the pack is in place, allowing your body to devote its energy to healing.

In conclusion, the addition of castor oil packs into your wellness routine can contribute significantly to your detoxification process. With their simple application yet multi-faceted benefits, castor oil packs are a natural, easy-to-integrate tool for overall health promotion.

38

Guidelines for Effectively Incorporating Hydration and Castor Oil Packs Into Your Routine

Establishing a routine that promotes hydration and detoxification through drinking water and using castor oil packs requires mindfulness. This chapter provides practical suggestions for integrating these elements seamlessly into your daily life.

Integrating Hydration: Drinking Water

1. **Start Your Day with a Glass of Water**: Consuming a glass of water upon waking up helps activate internal organs and jumpstart metabolic processes.
2. **Keep a Water Bottle With You**: Ensure you have access to water at all times by carrying a water bottle with you, regardless of location.
3. **Set Hydration Reminders**: Utilize reminders on your phone or smart device to help remember to drink water consistently throughout the day.
4. **Infuse Your Water**: Enhance your water by adding slices of fruit, veggies, or herbs, making it more enjoyable to consume.

Incorporating Castor Oil Packs for Detoxification

1. **Choose the Correct Position**: To maximize results, apply the pack to the liver and abdominal area while lying down comfortably.
2. **Set a Regular Schedule**: Depending on your body's response, utilize a castor oil pack 1-3 times a week for 1-2 hours to optimize benefits.
3. **Use a Heat Source**: Employ a mild heat source, such as a heating pad or hot water bottle, to improve the effectiveness of castor oil packs.
4. **Rest During Application**: Dedicate the duration of the application to rest and meditation, enabling your body to focus its energy on healing and detoxification.

XIII

Going Deeper with Detox: Coffee Enemas and Matcha Tea

39

Understanding Coffee Enemas for a Deep Detoxification Experience and the Beneficial Properties of Matcha Tea

Unveiling the realms of profound detoxification, coffee enemas and matcha tea emerge as powerful natural tools, with their unique roles in cleansing the body.

Coffee Enemas: The Deep Detox Tool

Coffee enemas roots trace back to ancient practices, championed for their pronounced detoxification abilities. Strategically targeted towards rigorous liver cleanse, the caffeine in coffee stimulates the liver to expedite its detoxification process, thereby eliciting a system-wide purification.

Utilizing Coffee Enemas

1. **Choose the Right Type of Coffee**: Opt for light roast organic coffee that's specifically designed for enemas.
2. **Preparation**: Prepare the coffee enema solution by brewing the coffee in purified water, letting it cool to body temperature.

3. **Application**: Ensure a comfortable and private space for the enema procedure. Utilize an enema kit to administer the coffee solution rectally. Retain the solution for about 15 minutes before releasing.

Matcha Tea: A Potent Detox Ally

Matcha tea, an exquisite variant of powdered green tea, blends in smoothly with any detox plan, given its rich antioxidant profile. It contains high concentrations of epigallocatechin gallate (EGCG), an antioxidant with significant detoxification potential, thereby aiding liver function and ramping up the body's detox capabilities.

Incorporating Matcha Tea in Your Routine

1. **Choose a Quality Product**: Invest in a high-quality, certified organic matcha to ensure you receive all beneficial properties.
2. **Prepare Matcha Tea**: Use a bamboo whisk to blend a teaspoon of matcha powder with hot (not boiling) water until frothy.
3. **Consumption**: Enjoy matcha tea on its own or as a part of your smoothies or lattes.

In conclusion, implementing coffee enemas and matcha tea into your wellness routine paves the path to deep detoxification, encompassing more than just physical cleansing but holistic rejuvenation.

40

Safe Practices While Undertaking Coffee Enemas and Matcha Tea

As you delve deeper into the world of detoxification with coffee enemas and matcha tea, it's crucial to undertake these practices safely. In this chapter, the focus is on illustrating the safe practices when embarking on these detox methods.

Coffee Enemas: Safe Practices

The procedure of coffee enemas, while beneficial, can pose certain risks if not done correctly. Here are some safety tips to follow:

1. **Type of Coffee**: Only use organic, light roast coffee specifically designed for enemas.
2. **Cleanliness**: Maintain high hygiene standards to prevent the risk of infections. Always thoroughly clean the enema equipment before and after use.
3. **Position**: Lie on your right side during the enema to facilitate the coffee reaching the liver more readily.
4. **Don't Rush**: Allow yourself plenty of time to relax both during and after the enema.

Matcha Tea: Safe Practices

Matcha tea, while potent and beneficial, should still be consumed responsibly. Here are some safety tips:

1. **Quality Matters**: Always choose high-quality, certified organic matcha powder to avoid exposure to pesticides or other harmful residues.
2. **Serving Size**: Abide by the rule of moderation. Limit your intake to one or two cups a day to avoid excessive caffeine or antioxidant intake.
3. **Consume with a Meal**: To maximize its absorption and limit potential side-effects, it's a good idea to consume matcha tea with your meal.

Detoxification using methods such as coffee enemas and matcha tea can contribute substantially to a profound cleanse. However, harnessing their benefits while ensuring safety reflects responsible practice, which is vital to sustainable wellness.

41

Pairing Coffee Enemas and Matcha Tea for Heightened Wellness Results

Combining coffee enemas with matcha tea intake can offer comprehensive wellness advantages, propelling you further in your detoxification journey. This chapter explores how to effectively pair these powerful tools for optimal wellness results.

Perfecting the Pair: Coffee Enemas and Matcha Tea

1. **Timing is Essential**: Start your day with a coffee enema to invigorate liver detoxification, followed by replenishment with a wholesome breakfast. Enjoy a cup of matcha tea later in the morning or early afternoon to maintain the detoxification momentum throughout the day.
2. **Consistency Yields Results**: Depending on your body's tolerance, aim to undertake a coffee enema 1–3 times a week. Incorporate a daily regimen of matcha tea to consistently promote detoxification.
3. **Listen to Your Body**: Pay attention to how your body responds to this pairing. Adjust frequency and portion size of both procedures as needed.
4. **Pair With a Balanced Diet**: A diet rich in fiber, fats, and protein can help support the detoxification process.

Unleashing Synergistic Benefits

When combined, the accelerated detoxification from coffee enemas and the antioxidant strength of matcha tea can create a powerful wellness synergy, amplifying their individual benefits. This includes enhanced liver function, increased toxin elimination, stimulated metabolism, improved digestion, and a boost in overall vitality.

The interplay of coffee enemas and matcha tea in a detox regimen layers on a potent detoxifying agenda, adopting a heightened path to holistic wellbeing.

XIV

Beyond Physical Aspects: Spiritual Detoxification

42

Introducing Spiritual Detoxification as a Vital Part of The Ruth Diet

As our exploration of The Ruth Diet continues, a shift from the physical to the intangible is initiated, emphasizing the prominence of spiritual detoxification in the pursuit of overall wellbeing. Punctuating our physical detoxification practices with spiritual wellness rituals, we aim to carve a holistic wellness trajectory that seamlessly combines the physical, mental, and spiritual elements of health.

Delving Deeper Into Spiritual Detoxification

Spiritual detoxification extends beyond the thresholds of our physical beings, exploring the less tangible but equally vital space of our spiritual selves. This practice spotlights the necessity to purge our minds and souls of persistent negative energies, emotional baggage, and mental chaos to set free a beaming stream of positivity, tranquility, and inner harmony.

Further Integrating Spiritual Detox into The Ruth Diet

In the spirit of embracing a well-rounded wellness approach, The Ruth Diet sees the potential in not only catering to bodily health but also nurturing spiritual tranquility. Let's delve further into strategic ways to incorporate spiritual detoxification:

- **Deep Meditation**: While we recognize daily meditation as crucial, it's equally important to occasionally engage in more profound, prolonged meditative sessions that facilitate deeper exploration of your psyche.
- **Focused Gratitude Practice**: Beyond regular note-taking, try to externalize your gratitude more openly, which could involve sharing your gratitude in conversations or displaying elements that symbolize your reasons for gratitude.
- **Advanced Yoga Practices**: Progress beyond basic yoga postures and invest in learning more complex poses and sequences that further connect the mind, body, and spirit.
- **Deeper Nature Connection**: Extend beyond passive time in nature to more immersive experiences. This could involve activities like hiking, forest bathing, or even camping trips to profoundly connect with nature.
- **Extended Detoxification Rituals**: Supplement standard practices like sage smudging or Epsom salt baths with spiritual retreats or engaging in structured spiritual cleansing programs.

By fusing the potent detox capabilities of practices like coffee enemas and matcha tea with robust spiritual practices, The Ruth Diet proposes a pathway to wellness that's truly comprehensive, harmonizing physical benefits with spiritual prosperity.

43

Practical Exercises and Routines for Spiritual Rejuvenation

The journey towards spiritual detoxification goes beyond understanding the principles. The most significant impact occurs when we can put the knowledge gained into practice. This chapter introduces practical exercises and routines that can be incorporated into your day-to-day life to foster spiritual rejuvenation.

Practical Spiritual Exercises

Transform your abstract understanding of spirituality into concrete actions through the following:

1. **Mindful Breathing**: Conscious mindful breathing can help tune mind-body connection and promote tranquility. You could start with five minutes of focused breathing every morning.
2. **Meditation Journal**: Documenting your meditation insights can deepen your self-awareness and provide a reference point for reflection.
3. **Gratitude Jar**: Daily write down something you're thankful for on a slip of paper and place it into a jar to visually represent your ongoing gratitude practice. Empty and read the notes each month, recapitulating

the abundant positivity in your life.

Routines for Spiritual Rejuvenation

Developing a comprehensive routine is key to maintaining consistent spiritual wellness:

1. **Morning Ritual**: Create a routine that includes meditative practices, yoga, and a hearty, nourishing breakfast.
2. **Scheduled Downtime**: Designate periods throughout your day for mental rest—pockets of time spent in nature, reading a book, or simply in quiet reflection.
3. **Evening Wind-down**: End the day with a combination of gentle stretching, journaling, and a relaxation practice such as aromatherapy or a warm bath.

Void of any refined sugars, artificial additives, The Ruth Diet provides comprehensive direction to pairing coffee enemas, matcha tea, and other sophisticated practices to rejuvenate not just the physical but also the spiritual dimension of human wellness.

44

Potential Outcomes of Integrating Spiritual Detoxification

As we continue to navigate the intricacies of spiritual detoxification, it's imperative to illuminate the prospects that underline the integration of these practices into our lives. This chapter not only outlines the potential benefits of adopting a spiritual detoxification route consistent with The Ruth Diet principles, but also broadens the picture to include more profound effects of such an integrated wellness approach.

Augmented Emotional Balance

Spiritual detoxification, by focusing on the purging of negative energies and emotions, can disproportionately enhance emotional stability. You could manifest fewer incidents of emotional volatility, fostering an equilibrated emotional state that contributes to happiness and peaceful existence.

Enriched Personal Integrity

Personal integrity stems from consistent alignment between your words and actions. Spiritual detoxification could encourage such alignment by increasing self-awareness and clarity about your personal values.

Longevity and Improved Quality of Life

Integrating physical and spiritual detoxification practices may potentially enhance longevity and the overall quality of life. As stress management improves and the immune response strengthens, it may result in a healthier, more vibrant existence punctuated with fewer health problems.

Better Decision Making

Spiritual detoxification could potentially hone your decision-making abilities. With a clearer mind and greater understanding and acceptance of personal values, you are likely to make more informed and aligned life choices.

Improved Connection with Nature and the Universe

Through the process of spiritual detoxification, you might find an enhanced sense of connection to nature and the universe at large. Understanding the interconnectedness of life can lead to profound experiences of awe and wonder, heightening ones sense of spiritual wellbeing.

The potential upshots of spiritual detoxification extend far beyond the obvious rejuvenation of the soul. They represent fragments of a mosaic foundation underpinning holistic wellbeing that encompasses all facets of wellness, physical, mental, emotional, and spiritual as envisioned by The Ruth Diet.

XV

Soul Cleanse: Love and Forgiveness

45

Essential Guidelines for Practicing Self-love and Forgiveness as a Part of Spiritual Detoxification

Plumbing deeper into the realms of self-love and forgiveness as prominent elements of spiritual detoxification, we foster an environment of acceptance and positive energy that is an incubator for spiritual growth. This extension of the chapter offers a deeper insight into practical exercises and mental shifts that support self-love and forgiveness within the framework of spiritual detoxification.

Amplifying the Power of Self-Love

Enriching the repository of self-love practices can foster deeper personal connections and improved self-image. Further strategies might include:

- **Embrace Solitude**: Grant yourself the license to enjoy solitude. Precious time spent alone in reflection provides an opportunity to connect with your inner self and bolster self-appreciation.
- **Affirmative Self-Talk**: Cultivate a habit of positive self-talk. Replace self-criticism with affirmations that uplift and validate your worth.

- **Manifest Gratitude**: Implement a daily gratitude practice. Appreciating instead of complaining can foster a profound shift towards self-love.
- **Seek Professional Help When Needed**: It's proactive and self-loving to engage professional help if emotional issues become overwhelming. Therapists and counselors can provide tools and techniques for healthier mental patterns.

Multi-Faceted Aspect of Forgiveness

Mature growth in the art of forgiving can help unblock energy pathways, ushering in peace and contentment. Here's how you can deepen your understanding and practice of forgiveness:

- **Understand Human Fallibility**: Recognize that everyone, including yourself, is susceptible to errors. This understanding promotes an environment ripe for forgiveness.
- **Detach Forgiveness from Reconciliation**: Understand that forgiveness is an internal process, essentially independent of the perpetrator's reaction or relationship status.
- **Utilize Meditation and Mindfulness**: Techniques such as lovingkindness meditation can encourage a forgiving mindset.
- **Seek Guidance**: If the pain of past wounds inhibits the process of forgiveness, seeking help from a counselor or spiritual guide could be beneficial.

In deepening our practice of self-love and forgiveness, we continuously detoxify our souls of negativity, making way for invigorating and positive energy. Integrating these enhanced guidelines into your spiritual detoxification regimen can significantly amplify your journey towards holistic wellbeing, as proposed by the fundamental principles of The Ruth Diet.

46

Relevant Exercises and Reflections to Follow for Soul Cleanse: Love and Forgiveness

Transitioning from theoretical approaches to actionable exercises, this chapter introduces practical methods to promote self-love and forgiveness within your spiritual detox regimen. By incorporating these targeted exercises into your daily routine, you can deeply nurture the healing power of love and forgiveness.

Exercises to Boost Self-Love

The following activities encourage self-love and compassion:

1. **Mirror Work**: Stand in front of the mirror, making eye contact with your reflection. Speak positive affirmations aloud, such as "I am worthy," "I am enough," and "I am loved."
2. **Journaling**: Dedicate a journal to celebrating your strengths and achievements. Revisit and add to this journal regularly to stay mindful of your unique abilities.
3. **Self-Compassion Visualization**: Close your eyes and visualize yourself

surrounded by warmth, love, and nurturing energy. Internalize this sensation and carry it with you as you go about your day.

4. **Create a Self-Love Ritual**: Design a daily regimen that prioritizes self-care, such as a warm bath, mindfulness meditation, or reading affirming literature.

Exercises to Foster Forgiveness

These practices support the cultivation of forgiveness:

1. **Forgiveness Letter**: Write a letter to yourself or others expressing your intention to forgive. This process releases the burden of pain and negative emotions and helps pave the road to healing.
2. **Empathy Activation**: Place yourself in the shoes of the person who wronged you. Reflect on their possible struggles and intentions to broaden your capacity for forgiveness.
3. **Forgiveness Meditation**: Practice guided forgiveness meditations consistently. These meditations walk you through the process of releasing pain, embracing forgiveness, and shifting your mindset.
4. **The Three R's Exercise**: In a quiet space, repeat these three phrases: "Recognize the pain," "Release the grudge," and "Realign with peace." Repeating these intentions can eventually alleviate the negative hold of past hurts.

By marking the transition from theory to practice with these targeted exercises, you can passionately pursue a path of self-love and forgiveness. Implementing these activities within your spiritual detoxification routine can profoundly influence your journey towards holistic wellbeing as envisioned by The Ruth Diet.

47

Stories of Individuals Who've Undergone Soul Transformation Through These Practices

This expanded chapter delves deeper into the awe-inspiring journeys of Melissa, Jackson, and Lily, providing greater insight into their transformation through self-love and forgiveness practices.

Melissa: Finding Self-Love

As a single mother, Melissa experienced countless moments of self-doubt and self-neglect. Exhausted, she sought solace and strength in The Ruth Diet principles. As she implemented mirror work exercises, she began verbalizing the self-love she had been denying herself. Each affirmation dismantled a brick in the fortress she'd built, and soon, her confidence soared. The words of self-appreciation resonated deep within her, fueling her determination.

Journaling became a sanctuary for Melissa, where she documented her deepest thoughts and celebrated her accomplishments. Over time, gratitude and self-awareness emerged; she recognized her own perseverance and ability to provide for her child.

Redefining self-love, Melissa prioritized self-care and found solace in her newfound confidence. With renewed vigor, she pursued her dreams and provided a stable and loving environment for her child.

Jackson: The Power of Forgiveness

Haunted by memories, Jackson often found himself consumed by resentment. On his journey of healing, he discovered the power of forgiveness. The act of writing a forgiveness letter was transformative, setting him on a path to emotional recovery.

With the empathy activation exercise, Jackson began to understand his comrade's motives and position. This understanding opened a door towards compassion, helping him accept the past without resentment. Releasing the burden of bitterness, Jackson experienced a newfound sense of freedom and inner peace.

Embracing forgiveness, he now encourages others in similar situations to seek solace in the healing power of forgiveness.

Lily: From Self-Loathing to Self-Love

Lily's journey from self-loathing to self-love was fraught with challenges, as she battled an eating disorder that eroded her sense of self-worth. Committed to change, she turned to visualization exercises, envisioning warmth and nurturing energy enveloping her. This warmth rooted itself within her as she connected deeply with her inner self, fostering self-love day by day.

Moreover, Lily adopted self-compassion meditation, embracing the practice wholeheartedly. She started to discard the harsh judgments she held towards her body and her disorder, replacing them with love and acceptance.

As Lily's capacity for self-love expanded, her recovery from the eating disorder accelerated. She gained the emotional strength required to reclaim control of her life, embracing all aspects of herself, both strengths and weaknesses.

In these stories, the power of self-love and forgiveness practices is palpable. Each narrative is a glowing testament to the immeasurable potential of these practices to create radical soul transformation.

XVI

Cases of Transformation: Stories from the Ruth Diet Alumni

48

Cases of Transformation: Stories from The Ruth Diet Alumni

This chapter shines a spotlight on the remarkable life transformations experienced by several individuals who devoted thirty days a year to practicing The Ruth Diet. The personal journeys of Brian, Sarah, Adam, and Naomi are testament to the immense healing potential of this regimen.

Brian: Finding Balance

As a devoted lawyer often buried in a surmounting pile of work, Brian grappled with stress and an impaired work-life balance. Immersing himself in The Ruth Diet practices for thirty dedicated days each year instigated a profound shift in his outlook. He began to cultivate inner peace, leading to balance in all spheres of life. The tension around him seemed to dissolve, paving the way for blossoming relationships and a significant reduction in professional stress. The elusive equilibrium that seemed unreachable was now part of his everyday life.

Sarah: Embracing Self-Love

Sarah spent her life in service as a compassionate nurse, frequently placing the needs of others above her own. Her decision to dedicate a month to The Ruth Diet was initially met with hesitation. However, this investment bore fruit as she discovered a deep sense of self-love that rejuvenated her perspective on life. While she continued to care for others, she realized the importance of prioritizing herself and her wellbeing—an often neglected aspect of her nurturing profession.

Adam: The Road to Forgiveness

Adam's life was tainted with resentment, a result of personal betrayals he had endured over the years. Committing to a month of The Ruth Diet presented him with a powerful tool—forgiveness. He was able to displace the bitterness he once harbored, setting off a healing process that culminated in unprecedented reconciliation with those he once considered his adversaries.

Naomi: From Anxiety to Calm

Naomi, perpetually anxious by nature, found her daily life governed by overwhelming stress. However, the transformation after immersing herself in The Ruth Diet for thirty days was palpable. She experienced tranquility and a sense of calm that she had long deemed unattainable. The practices of this regimen guided her towards mindfulness, remarkably reducing her anxiety levels and fostering a peaceful inner world.

These personal journeys underscore that embracing The Ruth Diet can instigate significant transformations, be it achieving balance, cultivating self-love, embarking on the path to forgiveness, or transitioning from anxiety to calm. They are a testament to the profound changes that dedication and commitment can bring about in one's life.

49

Varied Testimonials: Reflecting Different Challenges and Victories

This enlightening chapter presents a diverse range of testimonials, each echoing distinct challenges overcome and victories achieved through the devotion to The Ruth Diet practices.

Alex: Overcoming Grief

Alec, in the throes of deep grief following the loss of his partner, found courage and healing through the practices of The Ruth Diet. Over time, Alex found strength to navigate through his grief, cherishing the love he'd shared without being bound by loss.

Bella: Breaking Free from Addiction

Bella, trapped in the vicious cycle of addiction, saw hope through The Ruth Diet. With disciplined practice, she managed to shatter her chains of dependency, freeing herself from the shackles of addiction and embracing a fresh start.

Carlos: Turning Anger into Compassion

Carlos was a hot-tempered individual who often let anger cloud his judgment. However, after practicing The Ruth Diet, he experienced a radical transformation, managing to turn his anger into compassion, thereby improving his relationships and overall quality of life.

Donna: Overcoming Chronic Stress

Donna, engulfed by chronic stress due to her demanding career, found solace in The Ruth Diet practices. Now, she effectively manages her stress, resulting in improved mental health and productivity at work.

Eric: Conquering Fear of Failure

Eric always wrestled with crippling fear of failure. However, by focusing on the principles of The Ruth Diet, he managed to redefine his perception of success and failure, nurturing a growth mindset that allowed him to face life's challenges confidently.

These varied testimonials echo different challenges and victories, illuminating the transformative power of The Ruth Diet. Each journey of transformation serves as an inspiration to those embarking on their path of emotional healing and personal growth.

50

Revelations and Insights: Inspiring New Participants

The extended chapter constitutes a compendium of deeply insightful teachings and profound revelations, accrued by alumni of The Ruth Diet. These narratives serve as a lighthouse guiding new participants embarking on their personal journey towards transformation.

The Power of Consistency

Alumni earnestly stress the compelling significance of consistent practice, irrespective of how overwhelming the challenges or emotions might appear. They extol the virtues of daily dedication which, like a patient gardener, eventually leads to a robust tree of personal growth. The constancy they followed played a significant role in their transformation, unveiling the importance of nurturing a habit consistently.

Trusting the Process

Experienced adherents of The Ruth Diet underscore unequivocally the imperative to have faith in the process. With patience and resilience, they traversed the path when visible progress refused to mirror their efforts. Their surrender to the transformative force of The Ruth Diet yielded astonishing results, positioning new participants to reap the comprehensive benefits of this therapeutic practice.

The Importance of Self-Reflection

Reflection, as translated eloquently by the alumni, appeared as a key contributor to their personal growth. This informed introspection did not stem from spontaneous bursts of contemplation but was woven into their daily practice. Engaging in frequent self-assessment, they unravelled deep-seated patterns, destructive choices, and inhibitive beliefs that ostensibly marred their growth trajectory. Equipped with these elucidated insights, new participants are incited to dig deeper and venture onto the path of self-discovery in earnest.

Embracing Vulnerability

The concept of vulnerability, often wrapped in fear and misunderstanding, is warmly endorsed by The Ruth Diet's seasoned participants. They testify to the profound healing and empowered self-expression born out of embracing vulnerability. The courage to cast aside facades and confront fears led to enriched relationships and profound self-discovery. The alumni's transformative experiences serve to reassure and inspire new participants to embrace their vulnerability without apprehension.

Celebrating Victories

In conclusion, the alumni of The Ruth Diet impart the unsaid wisdom of recognizing and rejoicing in personal achievements, irrespective of their apparent magnitude. A single step of progress, a moment of self-revelation, or a conquered weakness are victories worthy of celebration. This acknowledgement of personal victories seeds positive momentum and fuels the constantly evolving cycle of growth and transformation.

XVII

Turn Back Time: Navigating the Final Step

51

An Overview of The Ruth Diet: Practical Advice for the Rejuvenating Journey

This chapter serves as an exhaustive guide to The Ruth Diet, offering indispensable advice for those prepared to embark on this rejuvenating and transformative journey.

Understanding The Ruth Diet

The Ruth Diet transcends the average dietary regimen, focusing instead on optimizing physical, mental, and emotional well-being. It is rooted in the principles of stable nutrition, balanced activities, mindfulness, and self-love, paving the way for harmony, internal healing, and personal rebirth.

Starting The Journey

Venturing forth on The Ruth Diet journey requires commitment and readiness for a complete lifestyle overhaul. The path encompasses daily routines of mindful eating, exercising, meditative practices, and deliberate self-care, all essential to the program's success.

Practical Advice

Outlined below are several essential pieces of advice to kickstart this transformative and rejuvenating journey:

Stay Consistent: A regular routine is pivotal for facilitating lasting change. Consistency cultivates incremental progress that, over time, yields striking results.

Trust the Process: Initially, tangible outcomes may seem tenuous. Regardless, remember that each stride taken contributes to the metamorphosis. Place unwavering faith in The Ruth Diet's efficacy and the ongoing progress being accomplished.

Self-Reflection is Key: Dedicate time each day to introspective reflection, examining actions, thoughts, and emotions. Fostering self-awareness elucidates obstructive patterns that facilitate targeted adjustments in the regimen.

Embrace Vulnerability: Far from denoting weakness, vulnerability signals transcending borders and embracing growth. Befriend vulnerability to unlock deep emotional healing and substantial growth.

Celebrate Victories: Lastly, make a point to recognize and rejoice in progress at each stage, no matter how minor it appears. This practice nurtures positivity and propels further momentum.

Galvanized by these practical tips, individuals of all backgrounds can confidently set forth on the rejuvenating journey offered by The Ruth Diet. This path promises a life steeped in health, balance, and personal growth.

52

Addressing Common Challenges and Concerns

This chapter delves deeper into understanding and navigating the common challenges and concerns that participants might experience while traversing The Ruth Diet journey, offering valuable insights and solutions to guide them.

Understanding and Overcoming Challenges

Struggling with Consistency: Maintaining steadfastness is often difficult for many. Establishing a personalized routine that aligns with individual lifestyles and preferences encourages improved adherence to the regimen. In moments of difficulty, remembering the long-term goals and objectives offers motivation to stay on track.

Frustration from Slow Visible Progress: Discouragement may arise when perceivable progress appears lackluster. Emphasizing that transformation is an enduring process requiring time and patience is vital. Focusing regularly on the positive shifts, regardless of their magnitude, incites motivation and maintains inspiration.

Feeling Overwhelmed by New Habits: Incorporating novel habits into daily routines might initially be intimidating. Ease into The Ruth Diet by initiating small, manageable changes, progressively integrating more intricate habits as the journey unfolds.

Addressing Concerns

Concern about Dietary Restrictions: The Ruth Diet emphasizes a healthier lifestyle, rather than restrictions. It champions a well-rounded diet abundant in nutrients. Through diligent planning and preparation, adherents can make maintaining a balanced diet both effortless and enjoyable.

Worry Regarding Physical Activity Requirements: Physical activity remains fundamental to The Ruth Diet's success, but adopting this practice does not mandate intensive workout sessions. Embrace activities that inspire joy and enthusiasm—dancing, walking, or gardening, for example—to seamlessly incorporate physical exertion into daily life.

Apprehension about Mindfulness Practice: Mindfulness does not obligate participants to embark on extensive meditation sessions. Instead, it invites explorations of presence and gratitude for the current moment. Commence the journey towards mindfulness by dedicating a few moments daily to concentrated breathing.

Equipped with these insights and strategies, participants can effectively confront and triumph over the challenges that might arise during their transformative Ruth Diet journey.

53

Tips and Tricks for a Successful Completion

This chapter delivers a collection of useful tips and tricks designed to steer participants towards successfully completing The Ruth Diet journey.

Championing Consistency

Ensure consistency by establishing a routine that doesn't feel burdensome but inspiring instead. Tailor the regimen to suit individual preferences and existing schedules. Small, manageable steps are more likely to culminate in large, long-term transformations.

Embracing Patience

Rome wasn't built in a day and personal transformation certainly isn't either. Embrace patience and celebrate every small stride forward. Recognize that every step, no matter its extent, brings you closer to your goals.

Mindfulness: The Secret Ingredient

Mindfulness is not just a practice, it's a lifestyle. Incorporate it into everyday life activities—eating, walking, or even doing chores. Engage all the senses, savor the moment, and observe the myriad alterations it brings about.

Body Love: Your Most Powerful Tool

Show your body love by feeding it nutrient-rich foods, giving it ample rest, and engaging in regular physical activities. Recognize and appreciate your body's capabilities, focusing on strength and resilience rather than perceived shortcomings.

Share The Journey

The journey becomes easier, and at times even fun when shared with others. Form a support group or find a diet buddy who has embarked on a similar journey. Share experiences, achievements, and even setbacks, transforming them into collective learning experiences.

Making Setbacks Your Comeback

Undoubted, there will be moments of stumble and fall. However, every setback can be viewed as a setup for a grand comeback. Learn from the experience, tweak your strategy if needed, and keep moving forward with renewed determination.

These tips and tricks, when employed, hold the power to propel you towards successfully accomplishing The Ruth Diet journey.

XVIII

The Ruth Diet Promise: Vibrant Youth, Vitality, and Harmonious Living

54

outline

Chapter 12: The Ruth Diet Promise: Vibrant Youth, Vitality, and Harmonious Living

- Providing a perspective on the continuous growth and health journey post the diet

The Ruth Diet: Turning Back Time in 30 Days doesn't only guide the readers on a transformative journey, but equips them with knowledge and practices for lifelong health and youthfulness. The proposed diet amalgamates biblical wisdom, modern science, and wellness practices, transcending the mere concepts of diet into a full-fledged shift towards a healthier and rejuvenated lifestyle.

55

Ascribing The Ruth Diet's Holistic Approach to Wellness

This chapter expands on the comprehensive, holistic approach that The Ruth Diet brings to wellness, focusing not only on physical health but also integrating mental and emotional well-being for a harmonious life.

Harmonizing Body, Mind, and Soul

The Ruth Diet goes beyond mere dietary modifications and fitness alterations; it advocates for a pervasive fusion of wellness into every sphere of life. It demands synergy between the body, mind, and soul, encouraging the cultivation of a healthier, happier, and a progressively vibrant existence. Regular self-reflection exercises, as well as journaling about personal growth and transformations, can add depth to this experience.

Integrative Nutritional Approach

The Ruth Diet encourages a balanced intake of all major nutrients, avoiding undue asceticism or excess. It solidifies the understanding that a mindful and enjoyable connection with food is paramount in achieving optimal health and vitality. Apart from following the outlined nutritional guidelines, actively seeking out and trying healthy recipes can make the process far more enjoyable and sustainable.

A Celebration of Physical Activity

Physical activities, through the lens of The Ruth Diet, are not avenues of punishment, but forums for celebrating the body's potential. By nurturing an affinity towards physical activity as a habitual practice, it ingrains a profound appreciation for the body's abilities. Exploring a range of activities - from yoga to swimming to strength training - can help keep the routine exciting and thus more likely to be maintained.

Respecting the Power of Rest

The Ruth Diet comprehends and respects the power of restful downtime. It doesn't just emphasize the amount but also the quality of rest, allowing the body the necessary time for regeneration and growth. Implementing good sleep hygiene practices, for instance, establishing a consistent sleep schedule, can enhance the quality of rest received.

Building Mindfulness into the Daily Routine

The concept of mindfulness permeates beyond isolated practices or exercises. The Ruth Diet endorses incorporating mindfulness in routine daily activities, paving the way for the cultivation of presence and amplifying overall well-being. Practicing gratitude, for instance, can be a simple but powerful way to enhance mindfulness in daily life.

Connecting with Nature

Finally, The Ruth Diet extols the connection with nature as a crucial component of wellness. This principle fosters appreciation for nature's abundance and emphasizes our inherent place in the grand ecological scheme of life.

Regular activities which promote a connection with nature, such as gardening or hiking, can all be rewarding practices.

By cherishing these cornerstones, The Ruth Diet delivers a holistic, integrative approach to wellness, promising vibrant youth, vitality, and harmonious living.

56

Highlighting the Transformation It Offers to Body, Mind, and Spirit

This chapter underlines the transformative impact that The Ruth Diet promises, forming a trinity of significant changes in body, mind, and spirit.

Physical Transformation: Embrace a New Vigor

The Ruth Diet's holistic approach towards nutrition and physical activity empowers individuals to recognize and embrace their bodies' potential. It fosters weight maintenance, enhanced energy levels, and improved physical fitness, symbolizing a renewed vigor and vitality.

Mental Transformation: Nurture a Positive Mindset

The Ruth Diet doesn't simply stop at physical changes. The journey encompasses alterations in mental outlook, encompassing positivity, self-acceptance, and resilience. It cultivates a positive mindset, replacing self-deprecating thoughts with self-appreciation, leading to a nurturing and accepting attitude towards self.

Spiritual Transformation: Discover Inner Peace

Beyond the physical and mental realms, The Ruth Diet guides practitioners on a spiritual journey to discover inner tranquility. Through mindfulness practices and connection with nature, individuals uncover a deep sense of inner peace and meaningful connection with the universe.

A Triad of Transformations

The Ruth Diet isn't merely a diet or exercise routine, but a triad of transformative journeys. It brings about profound changes on physical, mental, and spiritual planes, making a powerful impact on overall quality of life.

Such transformations not only improve the individual's health and well-being but also influence their interactions with others, further spreading the positive vibes. And each day of continuous practice results in incremental improvements that affirm the power of The Ruth Diet's holistic approach.

Embrace The Ruth Diet and witness the transformative journey of body, mind, and spirit, moving closer to vibrant youth, vitality, and harmonious living.

57

Providing a Perspective on the Continuous Growth and Health Journey Post The Ruth Diet

In this chapter, we delve into the notion of continued personal growth and health trajectory even beyond the initial engagement with The Ruth Diet, emphasizing that the wellness journey is a lifelong pursuit.

An Ongoing Journey, Not a Destination

Embracing The Ruth Diet marks the beginning of an ongoing wellness journey rather than a finite mission. The learnings and practices imbibed during this period serve as a foundation for continued growth.

Maintaining Physical Vitality

The physical transformation inspired by The Ruth Diet sets the stage for a lifetime of holistic health. Maintaining an active lifestyle and mindful eating habits become ingrained habits, fostering a lifelong dedication to physical wellbeing.

Sustaining Mental Wellness

The Ruth Diet's mental wellness principles help build resilience and sustain a positive outlook on life. The practices introduced, such as mindfulness and self–compassion, cultivate an environment conducive to mental peace and growth.

Nurturing the Spiritual Connection

The spiritual connection established during The Ruth Diet journey doesn't cease post-diet. Instead, this newfound spiritual awareness serves as a compass for navigating life's ups and downs, fostering a sense of peace and purpose.

Turning Lessons into Lifestyle

The transition post The Ruth Diet isn't about ceasing the practices learned but about integrating them into one's lifestyle. From dietary habits to physical routines, mindfulness practices to spiritual explorations, every aspect of The Ruth Diet becomes a part of the journey to vibrant youth, vitality, and harmonious living.

By seeing The Ruth Diet as a stepping stone towards a lifetime of health and wellness, one can truly reap the benefits it promises, experiencing ongoing growth and continuous enhancement of well-being.

XIX

The Ruth Diet: Fertility Management

58

How Liquid Fasting, as Part of The Ruth Diet, Can Help Couples Get Pregnant

This chapter delves into the benefits of liquid fasting as an integral component of The Ruth Diet, specifically exploring how it may potentially help couples enhance their fertility and increase their chances of conceiving.

Liquid Fasting: An Essential Element of The Ruth Diet

Liquid fasting has attracted attention in recent years for its numerous health benefits. As part of The Ruth Diet's holistic approach to wellness, liquid fasting supports physical, mental, and emotional well-being, along with addressing fertility concerns for couples trying to conceive.

The Hormonal Connection

Liquid fasting can help regulate hormonal imbalances, a crucial factor affecting fertility in both men and women. By improving insulin sensitivity and lowering insulin levels, liquid fasting encourages hormonal harmony, fostering a suitable environment for conception.

Weight Management

Maintaining a healthy weight is essential for both male and female reproductive health. Liquid fasting, integrated into The Ruth Diet's guidelines, assists in weight management, creating a stronger foundation for overall fertility.

Reducing Inflammation and Oxidative Stress

One often-overlooked aspect of fertility is the role of inflammation and oxidative stress in impairing reproductive health. Liquid fasting exhibits anti-inflammatory and antioxidant effects, protecting cells—including reproductive cells—from damage, thereby fostering a healthier environment for conception.

Enhanced Emotional Balance

Fertility struggles can weigh heavily on couples emotionally. Liquid fasting, combined with The Ruth Diet's focus on mental well-being, helps maintain emotional balance throughout this journey. Liquid fasting may promote mental clarity and decrease stress levels, providing solid support during emotional ups and downs.

The Right Approach to Liquid Fasting

While liquid fasting provides potential benefits, it's essential to implement it responsibly and sustainably. Consult with a healthcare professional before incorporating liquid fasting into your health journey, ensuring it aligns with your unique needs and circumstances.

In conclusion, liquid fasting enhances The Ruth Diet by offering additional fertility-related benefits. Supporting hormonal health, weight management, inflammation reduction, and emotional balance, liquid fasting can potentially boost a couple's chances of conceiving, all within the framework of vibrant youth, vitality, and harmonious living.

59

Long-Term Fertility Management Post The Ruth Diet

In this chapter, we'll examine the ways of maintaining fertility health in the long term, beyond the immediate scope of The Ruth Diet.

Maintaining an Optimal Lifestyle

A continuous practice of the wellness habits nurtured during The Ruth Diet can positively influence long-term fertility health. Dietary choices, regular exercise, liquid fasting, and stress management are all valuable components of a lifestyle conducive to maintaining fertility.

Hormone Health

A balanced hormonal environment, fostered during The Ruth Diet, is essential for sustained fertility health. Regular check-ups, a balanced diet, enough sleep, and stress management practices can help in maintaining this delicate harmony.

Weight Management

Steady weight control, promoted by The Ruth Diet, can contribute to healthy reproductive systems for both genders. Consistent exercise and a balanced, nutrient-rich diet are key to maintaining weight in a healthy range.

Nutritional Support

Continual support for gestational health with a nutrient-dense diet is a key strategy post Ruth Diet. Consuming foods rich in fertility-supporting nutrients like folic acid, omega-3 fatty acids, and antioxidants can help nurture an environment conducive to conception and a healthy pregnancy.

Regular Health Check-ups

Routine health examinations play a significant role in identifying potential fertility-related problems early, allowing for the most effective interventions. Regular check-ups are crucial for sustaining reproductive health and managing fertility in the long term.

In conclusion, the journey to improved fertility extends far beyond the span of The Ruth Diet. By maintaining an optimal lifestyle, focusing on hormone health, keeping weight within a healthy range, consuming a nutrient-rich diet, and prioritizing regular health check-ups, couples can look forward to long-term fertility health management.

60

Emotional Well-Being and Its Impact on Fertility Post The Ruth Diet

This chapter delves into the importance of emotional well-being and examines its impact on fertility health, beyond the immediate scope of The Ruth Diet.

Emotional well-being: A Key to Sustained Fertility

Emotional health, often overlooked, plays a crucial role in maintaining long-term fertility health. Stress, anxiety, and depression can create hormonal imbalances that may interfere with reproductive health.

Mindfulness and Stress Management

Practices like mindfulness, meditation, and yoga serve as excellent tools for managing stress levels. Maintaining emotional well-being through these techniques can be beneficial for sustaining hormonal balance and overall fertility health.

Emotional Support Networks

Having strong emotional supports, such as partners, friends, family, or a support group, can help to manage emotional pressures that come with fertility journeys. Social support plays an integral role in managing psychological health and enhancing fertility outcomes.

Professional Mental Health Support

Professional help like counselling and psychotherapy can equip individuals with strategies to manage emotional stressors and related fertility concerns. These strategies can aid in maintaining and improving emotional wellness, thereby supporting a healthy fertility journey.

Holistic Approach to Emotional Well-being

A holistic approach to emotional health, integrating physical activities and nutrition, mindfulness, social support networks, and professional mental health services, can lead to balance and a sense of well-being, thereby enhancing fertility health.

In conclusion, emotional well-being and its appropriate management is a vital aspect of long-term fertility health. By incorporating stress management techniques, nurturing strong social networks, and seeking professional help when needed, couples can enhance their emotional health, thereby supporting their fertility journey in the long term.

XX

Pursuing Your Purpose

61

The Spiritual Journey of Ruth: Preparing to Meet Your 'Boaz'

This chapter uses the spiritual journey of Ruth and her act of washing her face to meet Boaz as a metaphor for preparing oneself to embrace one's purpose and ascend to the next level.

Ruth's Spiritual Journey: A Metaphoric Guide

The life of Ruth symbolizes a transformative spiritual journey that taught her the essence of faith, perseverance, and preparedness. This serves as a metaphorical guide for individuals to adopt similar traits to gear up for their 'Boaz'- their purpose or next level of existence.

Washing Your Face to Meet Boaz

In the biblical account, before going to meet Boaz, Ruth washed her face. This act can be depicted as a cleansing ritual, symbolizing a fresh start or preparing oneself for a new beginning - a compelling metaphor for personal transformation and readiness.

Embracing Your 'Boaz'- Your Purpose

Meeting Boaz represents embracing one's destiny or purpose. Every phase of your journey, including the trials and tribulations, prepare you for this critical meeting. This readiness is akin to Ruth's act of washing her face, signifying an enlightened and receptive state of mind, prepared for the gifts and challenges that your purpose may bring.

Washing away Doubts and Fears

Just as Ruth washed her face, metaphorically, washing your doubts and fears can prepare you for your 'Boaz'. This act signifies cleansing oneself from negative perceptions and anxieties that can hinder your progression towards your purpose.

The Spiritual Elevation

Ruth's story conveys the important message of patiently cultivating oneself for one's higher purpose. This spiritual journey allows for the shedding of self-doubt, fear, and negativity, thereby facilitating personal growth and elevation to the next level.

In conclusion, the spiritual journey of Ruth and her preparation act of washing her face to meet Boaz serves as a powerful metaphor for personal transformation. By cleansing our doubts and negative perceptions, we can better prepare ourselves to embrace our purpose, accelerating our progression to the next phase of our journey.

62

The Power of Consistent Renewal in Pursuit of Your Purpose

In this chapter, we'll explore the value of consistent renewal in the journey of discovering and working toward one's purpose, building on the metaphor of Ruth's spiritual journey.

Embracing the Cycle of Renewal

Just like Ruth washing her face, personal renewal is an essential aspect of self-growth and progress. Consistent renewal enables us to evolve and develop, adapting ourselves to changing circumstances and continually refining our pursuit of our purpose.

Reassessing Your Goals

An integral part of consistent renewal is periodically reassessing your goals and ensuring they still resonate with your purpose. This practice allows you to stay focused on your objectives while making any necessary adjustments for growth and change.

Continuous Learning

The journey of self-discovery demands a genuine commitment to learning at every stage. Be open to acquiring new skills, insights, and knowledge, as they can equip you better to pursue your passions and purpose more effectively.

Embracing Change

Transformation is inevitable in our journey toward our purpose. By embracing change, we can adapt ourselves to new situations and challenges, allowing personal growth to propel us ever closer to our goals.

Practicing Self-Reflection

Self-reflection is vital for personal progress. By regularly introspecting and analyzing our experiences, we can identify areas for improvement and foster self-awareness, in turn enabling us to make informed decisions related to our purpose.

Cultivating Resilience

A constant cycle of renewal requires resilience. Cultivate the ability to bounce back from setbacks and maintain a growth mindset that encourages learning from experiences, both successes and failures. This attitude will help maintain focus on the path toward your purpose.

In conclusion, consistent renewal is an ongoing process that plays a crucial role in keeping us on track for our life's purpose. By reassessing goals, learning continuously, embracing change, practicing self-reflection, and cultivating resilience, we can progress forward, just as Ruth's spiritual journey and transformation prepared her to meet Boaz and embrace her destiny.

63

Nurturing Mind, Body, and Spirit in Pursuing Your Purpose

This chapter discusses the significance of nurturing the mind, body, and spirit, creating an equilibrium to support our journey toward discovering and realizing our life's purpose.

Balancing the Mind

Achieving mental balance is essential for focusing our energies onto our purpose. Engaging in activities that develop cognitive skills, emotional intelligence, and mindfulness helps cultivate mental harmony and clarity.

Strategies to Balance the Mind

1. Consistent learning: Acquire new knowledge and skills to expand mental horizons and foster intellectual growth.
2. Mindfulness practices: Engage in meditation, deep breathing exercises, and journaling to enhance focus and self-awareness.
3. Positive affirmations: Employ positive self-talk and visualization to promote a healthier self-image and outlook.

Fortifying the Body

Physical well-being is intimately connected to our overall stability, including our ability to pursue our purpose. An active, nutritious, and balanced lifestyle can boost energy levels, enhancing our mental and emotional health.

Strategies to Fortify the Body

1. Regular exercise: Engage in physical activity to increase stamina, maintain a healthy weight, and reduce stress.
2. Nutritious diet: Consume a balanced, wholesome diet rich in vitamins, minerals, and essential nutrients.
3. Adequate sleep: Prioritize proper sleep hygiene to promote physical recovery, optimal brain function, and emotional equanimity.

Strengthening the Spirit

A resilient spirit plays a crucial role in maintaining focus and determination on our path toward our purpose. Cultivating spiritual fortitude can provide inner strength and guidance, enabling us to overcome a wide range of challenges.

Strategies to Strengthen the Spirit

1. Spiritual practices: Engage in prayer, meditation, or other spiritual activities tailored to your belief system to enhance inner peace, gratitude, and guidance.
2. Connecting to nature: Spend time in natural environments to encourage reflection and foster a sense of connection to the broader world.
3. Cultivate compassion: Focus on developing empathy and compassion toward oneself and others, promoting a positive and supportive atmosphere conducive to spiritual growth.

In conclusion, nurturing the mind, body, and spirit is a cornerstone of our pursuit of purpose. By adopting strategies that balance the mind, fortify the body, and strengthen the spirit, we empower ourselves to handle challenges, foster personal growth, and remain steadfast in our journey.

XXI

Liquid Soup Recipes

64

Cabbage Broth and Its Benefits

Cabbage broth is a nutritious and comforting liquid recipe that can provide numerous health benefits. In this chapter, we'll go over a simple cabbage broth recipe and discuss its potential advantages to one's well-being.

Cabbage Broth Recipe

Ingredients

- 1 medium-sized green cabbage, chopped
- 6 cups of water or vegetable broth
- 2 medium-sized carrots, chopped
- 1 onion, chopped
- 2 celery stalks, chopped
- 2 garlic cloves, minced
- 1/2 teaspoon black pepper
- Salt, to taste
- Optional: fresh herbs (such as parsley or cilantro) for garnishing

Instructions

1. Heat a large pot over medium heat, adding a splash of water or olive oil to sauté the onion and garlic until soft and fragrant.
2. Add the carrots and celery, sautéing for another 3-4 minutes, stirring occasionally.
3. Add the chopped cabbage to the pot, mixing well with other vegetables.
4. Pour in the water or vegetable broth, ensuring the cabbage is submerged.
5. Season with salt and black pepper, adjusting the taste accordingly.
6. Simmer the mixture over low heat for about 45-60 minutes, or until the cabbage and other vegetables are tender.
7. Optionally, strain the broth for a purer liquid or keep the vegetables intact for a more filling soup.
8. Garnish with fresh herbs and serve hot.

Benefits of Cabbage Broth

Cabbage broth offers a wealth of health benefits, ranging from weight loss support to improved digestion.

Rich in Nutrients

Cabbage is an excellent source of vitamins C and K, as well as essential minerals like potassium and manganese. The abundance of nutrients in cabbage broth boosts overall health and vitality.

Weight Loss Support

Cabbage broth is low in calories and high in fiber, making it a perfect choice for those looking to maintain or lose weight. Consuming cabbage broth can help you feel satiated, reducing excessive calorie intake.

Improved Digestion

Cabbage is a great source of dietary fiber, which can aid in regulating bowel movements and enhancing overall digestive health. A warm bowl of cabbage broth can provide gentle support to your digestive system.

Anti-inflammatory Properties

Cabbage contains powerful antioxidants and phytonutrients known to have anti-inflammatory effects. Consuming cabbage broth may help decrease inflammation, promoting overall well-being and boosting immunity.

Detoxification

Cabbage has detoxifying properties due to its high concentration of glucosi-nolates, which can help support the body's natural detoxification process. Regular consumption of cabbage broth may contribute to improved liver function and toxin elimination.

In conclusion, cabbage broth is a simple and wholesome liquid recipe that provides numerous health benefits. It is rich in essential nutrients, supports weight loss, improves digestion, reduces inflammation, and helps detoxify the body. Enjoying a warm bowl of this delicious broth can help strengthen your body and reinforce your overall well-being.

65

Liquid Recipes: Tomato Basil Soup and Its Benefits

Tomato basil soup is a classic, comforting liquid diet recipe that is not only low in calories but also packed with powerful nutrients. Let's explore a simple recipe for this soup and the associated health benefits.

Tomato Basil Soup Recipe

Ingredients

- 5 ripe tomatoes, peeled and diced
- 1 onion, chopped
- 3 cups of vegetable broth
- 1 cup of fresh basil leaves
- 3 cloves of garlic, minced
- 1 teaspoon of sugar (optional)
- 1/2 cup of low-fat milk or a dairy-free alternative
- Salt and pepper, to taste

Instructions

1. Sauté the onion and garlic in a large pot until they're softened and fragrant.
2. Add the tomatoes, cooking for approximately 10 minutes, or until they're thoroughly softened.
3. Pour in the vegetable broth and add basil leaves.
4. Allow the mixture to simmer for about 15-20 minutes.
5. After the soup has cooled slightly, blend it with an immersion blender until it's smooth. You could also use a regular blender, but remember to cool it enough to handle safely.
6. Return the soup to the heat and stir in the milk, adding salt, pepper, and sugar (if desired) to taste.
7. Serve the soup hot, garnished with a few fresh basil leaves if you like.

Benefits of Tomato Basil Soup

The tomato basil soup stands as a flavorful and nourishing meal option, providing multiple health benefits.

Rich in Vitamin C

Both tomatoes and basil are excellent sources of vitamin C, known for its immune-boosting properties. A single serving of this soup can provide a substantial portion of your daily vitamin C requirement.

Heart Health

Tomatoes are rich in lycopene, a compound associated with heart health. Regular consumption of tomato basil soup can therefore contribute to a healthier heart.

Bone Health

Basil contains vitamin K, which is essential for blood clotting and bone health. Incorporating this soup into your diet can aid your bone health.

Digestive Health

The fiber content from tomatoes can nourish the gut and aid digestion. A bowl of tomato basil soup can help maintain a healthy digestive system.

Weight Management

Tomato basil soup is low in calories but high in fiber, providing a satiating meal that can aid in weight management.

In conclusion, tomato basil soup is a wholesome, flavorful choice for a liquid diet. The mixture of tomatoes' richness and basil's fragrant aroma creates a soup that's not only delicious but also offers a wide array of health benefits.

66

Beet Ginger Soup and Its Benefits

Beet Ginger Soup is an invigorating option for a liquid recipe, boasting vibrant flavors and remarkable health benefits. Below is a simple recipe to prepare this nourishing soup at home and a summary of its health benefits.

Beet Ginger Soup Recipe

Ingredients

- 3 medium-sized beets, peeled and diced
- 1 tablespoon of fresh ginger, grated
- 1 onion, chopped
- 2 cloves of garlic, minced
- 4 cups of vegetable broth
- 1 tablespoon of olive oil
- Salt and pepper, to taste
- Optional: Fresh herbs (like parsley or celery leaves) for garnishing

Instructions

1. In a large pot, heat the olive oil, then sauté the onion and garlic until they become soft and aromatic.
2. Add the grated ginger and diced beets to the pot, and continue to cook for a few more minutes.
3. Pour the vegetable broth into the pot, covering the beetroot pieces.
4. Bring the mixture to a boil, then reduce the heat and let it simmer until the beetroot pieces are tender, which should take about 25-30 minutes.
5. After letting the soup cool slightly, blend the mixture using an immersion blender or a standalone blender, until it reaches a smooth consistency.
6. Season the soup with salt and pepper to taste.
7. Serve hot, garnished with fresh herbs if desired.

Benefits of Beet Ginger Soup

Beet Ginger Soup, besides being a delicious liquid diet option, brings along several health benefits.

High in Nutrients

Beets are packed with essential nutrients like fiber, folate, and vitamin C, while ginger boasts medicinal properties and provides vitamin B6 and magnesium.

Immune-Boosting

The antioxidants and immune-boosting properties of ginger coupled with the high vitamin C content in beets contribute to a stronger immune system.

Aids Digestion

Ginger is known to soothe the digestive system and help with digestion. The high fiber content in beets also aids in maintaining a healthy digestive system.

Heart Health

Beets are rich in nitrates that can improve heart health by reducing blood pressure and improving blood flow.

Detoxifying Properties

Both beets and ginger contain compounds that help detoxify the body and support liver health.

In conclusion, Beet Ginger Soup is a warm, comforting liquid diet option that is rich in essential nutrients and beneficial for health in many ways. Regular consumption can boost your immune system, aid digestion, improve heart health, and help detoxify your body.

67

Creamy Cauliflower Soup and Its Benefits

Creamy Cauliflower Soup is a delicious option for a liquid diet recipe, with an elegant, delicate taste and a full range of health benefits. Here is a simple recipe and a highlight of the numerous health advantages that this soup provides.

Creamy Cauliflower Soup Recipe

Ingredients

- 1 large cauliflower head, chopped into florets
- 1 onion, chopped
- 2 cloves of garlic, minced
- 4 cups of vegetable broth
- 1/2 cup of low-fat milk or a dairy-free alternative
- 1 tablespoon of olive oil
- Salt and pepper, to taste
- Optional: Fresh herbs (like parsley or chives) for garnishing

Instructions

1. In a large pot, heat the olive oil and then sauté the onion and garlic until they're soft and fragrant.
2. Add the cauliflower florets to the pot and cook for a few more minutes.
3. Pour in the vegetable broth, making sure the cauliflower is fully submerged, and then bring the mixture to a boil.
4. After it's boiling, reduce the heat and let it simmer until the cauliflower is tender, which should take about 15–20 minutes.
5. Once the soup has cooled a bit, blend it either using an immersion blender or a regular blender (make sure it's safely cooled) until it's smooth and creamy.
6. Stir in the milk, adding salt and pepper to your liking.
7. Serve warm, garnished with fresh herbs if desired.

Benefits of Creamy Cauliflower Soup

Creamy Cauliflower Soup, aside from being tastefully indulgent, provides an array of health benefits.

Nutrient-Rich

Cauliflower is high in essential nutrients like vitamins C, K, B6, and folate. It's also a good source of dietary fiber.

Boosts Immunity

The hefty amount of vitamin C in cauliflower helps to boost your immune system, enhancing your body's ability to ward off illnesses.

Bone Health

Vitamin K, found in abundance in cauliflower, contributes to bone health by aiding in calcium absorption and reducing urinary excretion of calcium.

Heart Health

The fiber in cauliflower helps to improve overall heart health by reducing bad LDL cholesterol levels and boosting good HDL cholesterol.

Aids Digestion

The dietary fibers in cauliflower can help maintain a healthy digestive system, preventing constipation and promoting regular bowel movements.

In conclusion, Creamy Cauliflower Soup serves as a satisfying and wholesome choice for a liquid diet. The creamy texture paired with its nutritional content and health benefits make it a win-win solution for those who prioritize both taste and wellness.

68

Spinach Broccoli Soup and Its Benefits

Spinach Broccoli Soup, packed with nutritious greens, is a notable liquid diet recipe that's both low in calories and high in nutritional value. Following is an easy-to-make Spinach Broccoli Soup recipe and an overview of its health benefits.

Spinach Broccoli Soup Recipe

Ingredients

- 1 medium-sized broccoli, chopped
- 2 cups of spinach leaves, washed
- 1 onion, chopped
- 2 cloves of garlic, minced
- 4 cups of vegetable broth
- 1 teaspoon of olive oil
- Salt and pepper, to taste
- Optional: Fresh herbs (such as parsley) for garnishing

Instructions

1. In a large pot, heat the olive oil and sauté the onion and garlic until soft and fragrant.
2. Add the chopped broccoli to the pot and cook for another few minutes.
3. Pour in the vegetable broth and bring it to a boil.
4. Once the mixture is boiling, reduce the heat and let it simmer until the broccoli is cooked, which usually takes about 15-20 minutes.
5. Add the spinach leaves and cook for another 2-3 minutes, or until the spinach has wilted.
6. Once everything is well-cooked, use an immersion blender to blend the soup to a smooth consistency. Alternatively, you can let it cool and blend it in a regular blender.
7. Season the soup with salt and pepper to taste.
8. Garnish with fresh herbs and serve hot.

Benefits of Spinach Broccoli Soup

The Spinach Broccoli Soup is a healthy concoction that offers multiple health benefits.

Nutrient-Dense

Both spinach and broccoli are rich in essential nutrients like vitamins A, C, K, and B vitamins, as well as minerals like iron, calcium, and potassium. This makes the soup a nutritious choice.

Boosts Immune System

Given its high vitamin A and C content, Spinach Broccoli Soup can help strengthen your immune system and fight off different types of infections and diseases.

Bone Health

The presence of vitamin K in both spinach and broccoli contributes to bone health by aiding calcium absorption and blood clotting.

Heart Health

The fiber and antioxidants found in spinach and broccoli can help lower cholesterol levels, thereby promoting heart health.

Weight Loss

This soup is low in calories yet high in fiber, which can help you feel fuller and reduce unnecessary calorie intake, aiding in weight management.

Thus, Spinach Broccoli Soup stands as a great liquid diet option due to its nutrient-density and health benefits. Regular consumption of this soup can contribute to overall wellbeing, boosting immunity, promoting bone and heart health, and aiding digestion and weight loss.

69

Pumpkin Soup and Its Benefits

Pumpkin soup is a rich, creamy, and satisfying meal that offers a wealth of nutritional benefits. In this chapter, we delve into an easy-to-follow pumpkin soup recipe and explore its health advantages.

Pumpkin Soup Recipe

Ingredients

- 1 small pumpkin, peeled and diced
- 1 onion, chopped
- 2 garlic cloves, minced
- 4 cups of vegetable broth
- 1 cup of coconut milk
- 1/2 teaspoon of cinnamon
- 1/2 teaspoon of nutmeg
- Salt and pepper, to taste
- Optional: Pumpkin seeds for garnishing

Instructions

1. In a large pot, sauté the onion and garlic until they're soft and fragrant.
2. Add the diced pumpkin to the pot and sauté for a few more minutes.
3. Pour the vegetable broth into the pot, ensuring the pumpkin is fully submerged. Bring the mixture to a boil.
4. Reduce the heat and allow it to simmer until the pumpkin is tender, approximately 20–25 minutes.
5. Once the pumpkin is cooked, blend the mixture using an immersion blender until it reaches a smooth consistency. Alternatively, you can use a conventional blender, but ensure the soup is cool enough to handle safely.
6. Stir in the coconut milk, cinnamon, and nutmeg. Season it with salt and pepper to taste.
7. Simmer the mixture for a few more minutes, stirring it occasionally.
8. Garnish with pumpkin seeds (optional) and serve it hot.

Benefits of Pumpkin Soup

Pumpkin soup is not only flavorful but also packed with essential nutrients.

High Nutritional Value

Pumpkin is a rich source of vitamins A, C, E, and several B vitamins. It's also packed with minerals like potassium, copper, and manganese.

Boosts Immune System

With its high vitamin C content, pumpkin soup can help boost your immune system, thereby helping to fight off various diseases.

Digestive Health

Pumpkin is a good source of fiber, which aids in digestion. Consuming pumpkin soup can therefore help support a healthy digestive system.

Healthy Eyes

Pumpkin is rich in beta-carotene, which is converted into vitamin A in the body. Vitamin A is essential for eye health and can contribute to protecting your vision.

Weight Loss

Pumpkin soup is low in calories and high in fiber, which can help you feel fuller for longer, ultimately aiding in weight loss.

In conclusion, pumpkin soup is a delicious and nutritious liquid recipe, suitable for those seeking both taste and health benefits. Regular consumption can contribute to improved immunity, digestive health, eye health, and could even aid weight loss.

XXII

Juicing recipes

70

Green Energy Booster and Its Benefits

The Green Energy Booster is a revitalizing and rejuvenating juicing recipe, packed with nutrient-dense fruits and vegetables. This wholesome and flavorful juice is easy to prepare and offers several health benefits.

Green Energy Booster Recipe

Ingredients

- 2 cups of kale leaves, washed
- 1 green apple, chopped
- 1 cucumber, sliced
- 1 celery stalk, chopped
- 1 small lemon, peeled and deseeded
- 1 small piece of ginger (approx. 1 inch), peeled
- Optional: A few mint leaves for extra freshness

Instructions

1. Wash all fruits and vegetables thoroughly.
2. Prepare your juicer, ensuring that all parts are clean and in working order.

3. Process the kale leaves, green apple, cucumber, celery stalk, lemon, and ginger through the juicer, one ingredient at a time.
4. If desired, add a few mint leaves to impart extra refreshing flavor.
5. Once complete, stir the juice well to ensure all components are fully mixed.
6. Pour the juice into a glass and enjoy immediately for the best taste and nutrient retention.

Benefits of Green Energy Booster

The Green Energy Booster juice offers a variety of health benefits due to its nutrient-rich ingredients.

Rich in Antioxidants

Ingredients like kale, green apple, celery, and lemon contain a myriad of antioxidants. These antioxidants help neutralize free radicals, reduce inflammation, and promote overall good health.

Boosts Energy Levels

The vitamins and minerals present in this juice, particularly B vitamins, vitamin C, and iron, can help increase energy levels and invigorate the body.

Supports Digestive Health

The presence of digestive aids, such as ginger, combined with the fiber content of fruits and vegetables, can help promote a healthier digestive system.

Immune System Support

The antioxidant and vitamin C content of the Green Energy Booster can help strengthen the immune system, offering added protection against various illnesses.

Skin Health

The juice's high vitamin A and C content can support skin health, keeping the skin hydrated and promoting a youthful appearance.

Heart Health

Ingredients like celery and cucumber contain nutrients beneficial for heart health, including potassium and magnesium, helping maintain a healthy blood pressure.

In conclusion, the Green Energy Booster juice is not only a delicious and refreshing drink but also a powerhouse of nutrients. Incorporating this detoxifying juice into your daily routine can contribute to overall good health, improved energy levels, better digestion, and enhanced immunity.

71

Sunshine Citrus Delight and Its Benefits

The Sunshine Citrus Delight is a vibrant and refreshing juicing recipe, featuring a delightful blend of citrus fruits and a dash of carrot sweetness. This invigorating and nutrition-packed juice is simple to prepare and has numerous health benefits.

Sunshine Citrus Delight Recipe

Ingredients

- 2 medium oranges, peeled and deseeded
- 1 medium grapefruit, peeled and deseeded
- 2 medium carrots, cleaned and chopped
- 1 small lemon, peeled and deseeded
- Optional: A touch of honey or a few drops of liquid stevia for added sweetness (if desired)

Instructions

1. Thoroughly wash and prepare the fruits and carrots.
2. Set up your juicer, ensuring all parts are clean and functioning properly.
3. Juice the oranges, grapefruit, carrots, and lemon one at a time, letting

their juices combine.

4. If desired, mix in honey or stevia to sweeten the final juice.
5. Stir the juice well to integrate all components thoroughly.
6. Pour your Sunshine Citrus Delight into a glass and enjoy right away to benefit from the maximum freshness and nutrient content.

Benefits of Sunshine Citrus Delight

The Sunshine Citrus Delight juice offers a variety of health benefits due to the abundance of vitamins and minerals found in its ingredients.

Rich in Vitamin C

Citrus fruits like oranges, grapefruits, and lemons are packed with vitamin C, which helps strengthen the immune system, support skin health, and aid in iron absorption.

Antioxidant Properties

The juice is abundant in antioxidants from the citrus fruits, promoting overall health by neutralizing free radicals and reducing inflammation.

Heart Health

Grapefruits in particular have been linked to improved heart health, including lower blood pressure and reduced risk of heart disease. Carrots also provide nutrients like potassium necessary for maintaining cardiovascular health.

Supports Healthy Vision

Carrots are rich in beta carotene, which converts into vitamin A in the body, and is essential for maintaining healthy vision and eye function.

Aids Digestion

The soluble fiber present in citrus fruits, in addition to the presence of vitamin A in carrots, can contribute to maintaining a healthy digestive system.

Better Hydration

The high water content of citrus fruits and carrots makes this juice a refreshing and hydrating choice.

In conclusion, the Sunshine Citrus Delight is a scrumptious and revitalizing drink, abundant in essential nutrients. Including this juice in your daily routine can positively impact your overall health, strengthen your immune system, support heart and digestive health, and maintain healthy vision.

72

Tropical Antioxidant Fusion and Its Benefits

The Tropical Antioxidant Fusion is a delicious and refreshing juicing recipe that combines a colorful mix of tropical fruits. This nutrient-dense, vibrant juice is simple to prepare and boasts of numerous health benefits.

Tropical Antioxidant Fusion Recipe

Ingredients

- 1 medium mango, peeled and pitted
- 1 cup of pineapple chunks
- 1 medium orange, peeled and deseeded
- 1 small piece of ginger (approx. 1 inch), peeled
- Optional: A squeeze of fresh lime juice for added tang

Instructions

1. Clean the fruits thoroughly and prepare them as directed.
2. Set up your juicer, ensuring all parts are clean and functioning properly.
3. Process the mango, pineapple, orange, and ginger through the juicer.
4. If desired, squeeze fresh lime juice into the finished product for an added zesty kick.

5. Stir the juice well to fully combine the flavors.
6. To enjoy the full burst of flavors and nutrients, pour the juice into a glass and drink it immediately after preparation.

Benefits of Tropical Antioxidant Fusion

The Tropical Antioxidant Fusion juice offers a range of health benefits due to the array of nutrients present in its ingredients.

Antioxidant Rich

Mango, pineapple, and orange are packed full of antioxidants, which help protect the body against disease, slow down aging, and promote overall good health.

Immune System Support

The vitamin C content from these fruits, particularly the orange, helps strengthen the immune system and increases the body's resistance to various diseases.

Digestive Health

Pineapple is renowned for its digestion-aiding enzyme bromelain. Likewise, mango and orange also have considerable fiber content which helps in maintaining a healthy gut.

Anti-Inflammatory

Both pineapple and ginger are well known for their anti-inflammatory properties. Regularly including these in your diet can help reduce inflammation in the body.

Eye Health

Mangoes are rich in vitamin A, which is essential for good vision and eye health. It also helps maintain healthy mucous membranes and skin.

Hydrating

The high water content of these tropical fruits makes this juice a wonderfully hydrating drink.

In conclusion, the Tropical Antioxidant Fusion is a healthy, nutrient-packed juice that not only tantalizes your taste buds but also nourishes your body. Enjoying this tropical delight can contribute to improved immune function, enhanced digestive health, reduced inflammation, and better eye health.

73

Beetroot Bliss and Its Benefits

The Beetroot Bliss is a nutritious and robust juicing recipe, packed with a powerful combination of root vegetables and fruits. This vibrant and earthy juice is straightforward to make and offers several health advantages.

Beetroot Bliss Recipe

Ingredients

- 2 medium-sized beetroots, peeled and chopped
- 2 large carrots, cleaned and chopped
- 1 apple, cored and sliced
- 1 small piece of ginger (approx. 1 inch), peeled
- 1 small lemon, peeled and deseeded
- Optional: A touch of honey to sweeten, if desired

Instructions

1. Clean all fruits and vegetables thoroughly.
2. Set up your juicer, verifying all parts are clean and operational.
3. Process beetroots, carrots, apple, ginger, and lemon through the juicer in turn, allowing their juices to combine.

4. If desired, add honey to the juice to enhance its sweetness.
5. Stir the juice vigorously to blend all the ingredients smoothly.
6. Serve the juice in a glass immediately for maximum freshness and to retain the most nutritive value.

Benefits of Beetroot Bliss

The Beetroot Bliss juice concoction offers an array of health benefits due to the nutritious fruits and vegetables it contains.

Improved Stamina

Beetroots are known to boost endurance and stamina, which can be especially beneficial for active individuals or athletes.

High Antioxidant Level

The ingredients in this juice, especially beets and apples, are packed with antioxidants that counteract oxidative stress and inflammation.

Heart Health

Beetroots and carrots both offer heart-protective benefits. They help to lower blood pressure and reduce the risk of heart disease.

Digestive Support

The fiber from apples and carrots, along with beetroot and ginger, aids digestion, making this juice a good choice for digestive health.

Enhanced Immunity

This juice delivers a robust blend of vitamins and minerals like vitamin C, vitamin A, potassium, and folate that helps strengthen the immune system.

Healthy Skin

The high mineral content in this juice, particularly from beets and carrots, promotes healthy and glowing skin.

In conclusion, the Beetroot Bliss is a great choice of juice for its earthy tones, nutrient richness, and versatility. This juice is a potent mix of health benefits right from bolstering your stamina to enhancing your skin health.

74

Berry Fresh Antioxidant Punch and Its Benefits

The Berry Fresh Antioxidant Punch is a delightful and refreshing juicing recipe, infused with a potent mix of berries and fruits. This vibrantly colored juice is easy to make and offers a spectrum of health benefits.

Berry Fresh Antioxidant Punch Recipe

Ingredients

- 1 cup of strawberries, hulled
- 1 cup of blueberries
- 1 medium apple, cored and sliced
- 1 small lemon, peeled and deseeded
- Optional: A few leaves of fresh mint for an extra layer of freshness

Instructions

1. Wash all fruits and mint leaves (if using) thoroughly.
2. Prepare your juicer, ensuring all parts are clean and functioning well.
3. Feed the strawberries, blueberries, apple, and lemon through the juicer,

allowing the juices to combine.

4. Optionally, add a few fresh mint leaves for an additional refreshing flavor.

5. Once done, stir the juice to fully mingle the flavors.

6. Serve the juice immediately in a glass to retain its taste and nutritious potency.

Benefits of Berry Fresh Antioxidant Punch

The Berry Fresh Antioxidant Punch juice delivers a spectrum of health benefits due to its nutrient-rich ingredients.

Antioxidant Powerhouse

Berries like strawberries and blueberries are well known for their high antioxidant content. These antioxidants counteract free radicals, promoting heart health, boosting brain health, and potentially preventing certain types of cancer.

Vitamin C Rich

Strawberries and lemons are abundant in vitamin C, playing a crucial role in boosting the immune system, enhancing skin health, and aiding iron absorption.

High in Fiber

Both the apple and the berries in this recipe are high in dietary fiber. Consuming foods high in fiber supports digestive health, aids in weight management, and promotes heart health.

Anti-Inflammatory Properties

Blueberries, in particular, have anti-inflammatory properties that can help fight inflammation in the body.

Hydrating and Refreshing

The high water content of the fruits used makes this juice a great hydration solution, particularly on hot days or after exercising.

In conclusion, the Berry Fresh Antioxidant Punch is a refreshing and healthful juice choice. It is loaded with vitamins, minerals, fiber, and antioxidants — making it a delicious and nutritious addition to any balanced diet.

75

Green Garden Goodness and Its Benefits

The Green Garden Goodness is a nutrient-rich and energizing juicing recipe, showcasing a vibrant blend of green vegetables and fruits. This refreshing juice is quite easy to whip up and offers an array of health benefits.

Green Garden Goodness Recipe

Ingredients

- 2 large cucumbers
- 2 cups of fresh spinach
- 2 green apples, cored and sliced
- 1 small piece of ginger (approx. 1 inch), peeled
- 1 small lime, peeled and deseeded
- Optional: A few mint leaves for additional freshness

Instructions

1. Wash all the ingredients thoroughly.
2. Ensure your juicer is clean and ready for use.
3. Juice the cucumbers, spinach, green apples, ginger, and lime sequentially, allowing their juices to combine.

4. Optionally, add a few mint leaves to enhance the cool, refreshing flavor.
5. Stir the juice well, ensuring all flavors have been incorporated.
6. For the most beneficial nutrients and flavors, serve the juice immediately.

Benefits of Green Garden Goodness

The Green Garden Goodness juice offers a spectrum of health benefits due to the nutrient-dense fruits and vegetables used in its preparation.

Rich in Vitamin K

Spinach and cucumbers are excellent sources of Vitamin K which is necessary for blood clotting and bone health.

Anti-Inflammatory Properties

The ginger in this juice is well known for its anti-inflammatory properties, which help to reduce inflammation within the body.

High in Fiber

Green apples are a good source of fiber. A diet high in fiber helps to regulate the digestive system and can also aid in weight management.

Hydrating and Refreshing

Cucumbers, being rich in water content, along with the refreshing flavor of lime and optional mint, makes this juice an excellent hydrating drink.

Detoxifying

The combination of cucumber, mint, and lime, makes this juice a great detoxifying agent.

Boosts Immunity

The vitamin C found in green apples and lime helps to promote overall health by boosting the immune system.

In conclusion, Green Garden Goodness is a smart choice for those looking to incorporate a healthy, refreshing, and nutrient-rich juice into their daily routine. It not only pleases the palate but also contributes towards good health.

XXIII

Conclusion

76

Conclusion

The journey we have embarked on has allowed us to delve deep into the benefits, deliciousness, and simplicity of incorporating juicing into our daily lives. We have seen how each ingredient contributes its unique flavors and nutrients to create invigorating recipes packed with holistic benefits.

From recipes that act as fuel to boosting body stamina with the Beetroot Bliss, to those that are antioxidant powerhouses like the Berry Fresh Antioxidant Punch, every juice offers an entirely different palette of flavors and health benefits. The Tropical Antioxidant Fusion and Green Garden Goodness have shown us the versatility of juicing in balancing enjoyable flavors with health-promoting ingredients.

Juices provide us with concentrated doses of vitamins, minerals, and antioxidants that can improve various aspects of our health. Apart from these, some recipes also offer powerful anti-inflammatory benefits, such as those found in the delicious Beetroot Bliss and Green Garden Goodness.

We have seen how these recipes not only facilitate better physical health but also help to enhance the quality of our daily living. Regular juicing can have visible effects on skin health, digestion, immune strength, and hydration levels, paving the way towards a healthier, fresher, and more vibrant lifestyle.

More importantly, the act of preparing these juices can become a mindful and rewarding daily ritual. The vibrant colors of fruits, the earthy tones of vegetables, and the fusion of flavors created from combining these produce items in various ways offer an opportunity to connect with nature's bounty, appreciate its benefits, and empower ourselves to make healthier choices.

In closing, this comprehensive guide was designed to inspire and facilitate a delightful juicing journey. One that enhances your health, satiates your taste buds, and elevates your overall wellbeing. Here's to venturing into a future where we make informed, deliberate choices about our nutrition, embracing a lifestyle that prioritizes wellness.

77

"Juicing to Revitalization: Concluding the Journey"

As we reach the end of this enlightening journey, we reflect on the valuable insights and knowledge gained through the exploration of juicing and its remarkable benefits. We have uncovered the power of blending fruits and vegetables into liquid gold, a treasure trove of nutrients that can transform our health and wellbeing. Each recipe in this book has demonstrated the diversity and versatility of juicing, opening new doors to taste and health alike.

From invigorating blends such as the Tropical Antioxidant Fusion to rejuvenating recipes like the Green Garden Goodness, every juice offers a unique combination of flavors and benefits. We have witnessed how juicing can boost vitality, support detoxification, strengthen the immune system, and more.

In turn, this guide has highlighted how juicing not only affects physical health but also influences the quality of our everyday lives. The regular consumption of fresh juices can lead to improvements in energy levels, mental clarity, and overall happiness. In a world that is increasingly driven by convenience and instant gratification, the discipline of juicing offers a rewarding, grounding ritual that reconnects us to the earth's natural richness.

Throughout these chapters, we have emphasized the importance of perseverance, creativity, and experimentation. Juicing need not be an unvarying routine, but rather an evolving journey full of exciting flavor combinations and health discoveries. By taking charge of our nutrition and paying close attention to the types of foods we consume, we enhance our understanding of our bodies and make more significant strides towards improved wellbeing.

In conclusion, this guide is an invitation to embrace the transformative power of juicing. It encourages us to nourish ourselves with nutrient-dense, delicious recipes that elevate our health and introduce us to new culinary horizons. May your juicing journey be a source of revitalization, rejuvenation, and renewal, and may the blends you create lead to a vibrant, flourishing life.